Pain Management
for Older Adults

Mission Statement

IASP brings together scientists, clinicians, health care providers, and policy makers to stimulate and support the study of pain and to translate that knowledge into improved pain relief worldwide. IASP Press publishes timely, high-quality, and reasonably priced books relating to pain research and treatment.

Pain Management for Older Adults

A Self-Help Guide

Editors

Thomas Hadjistavropoulos

Heather D. Hadjistavropoulos

Department of Psychology and Centre on Aging and Health, University of Regina, Regina, Saskatchewan, Canada

IASP PRESS® | SEATTLE

Library of Congress Cataloging-in-Publication Data

Pain management for older adults : a self-help guide / editors Thomas Hadjistavropoulos, Heather D. Hadjistavropoulos. p.cm.

This manual was written to address the needs and concerns of older adults who experience chronic pain. The book presents a self-help program developed by pain researchers and healthcare professionals. It includes information about pain-related topics and easy-to-follow techniques and strategies (including exercises) that show older adults how to better manage chronic pain. --Provided by publisher

Includes bibliographical references and index.

ISBN 978-0-931092-70-1 (softcover : alk. paper)

1. Pain in old age--Treatment--Popular works. I. Hadjistavropoulos, Thomas. II. Hadjistavropoulos, Heather D., 1967-

RB127.P3323528 2008

618.97'60472--dc22   2007037338

Text and cover design by Sarah Watson Design

Published by:

IASP Press®
International Association for the Study of Pain

111 Queen Anne Ave N, Suite 501

Seattle, WA 98109-4955, USA

Fax: 206-283-9403

www.iasp-pain.org

Printed in the United States of America

Table of Contents

Contributing Authors

B. Lynn Beattie, MD, FRCP(C)
   UBC Hospital, Vancouver, British Columbia, Canada

Stephanie Cook, MSc, RD
   Clinical Nutrition Services, Regina Qu'Appelle Health Region,
   Regina, Saskatchewan, Canada

Shannon Fuchs-Lacelle, PhD
   Wascana Rehabilitation Centre, Regina,
   Saskatchewan, Canada

Romayne Gallagher, MD, CCFP
   Head, Division of Residential Care, Providence Health Care,
   Vancouver, Canada

Heather D. Hadjistavropoulos, PhD, RD Psych
   Department of Psychology and Centre on Aging and Health,
   University of Regina, Regina, Saskatchewan, Canada

Thomas Hadjistavropoulos, PhD, RD Psych
   Department of Psychology and Centre on Aging and Health,
   University of Regina, Regina, Saskatchewan, Canada

Elizabeth Harrison, PhD, BPT
   School of Physical Therapy, University of Saskatchewan,
   Saskatoon, Saskatchewan, Canada

Sandra M. LeFort, PhD, RN
   School of Nursing, Memorial University of Newfoundland,
   St. John's, Newfoundland, Canada

Ronald R. Martin, PhD, RD Psych
   Faculty of Education, University of Regina, Regina,
   Saskatchewan, Canada

Robert McCulloch, PhD
   Saskatchewan Institute of Applied Science and Technology,
   Saskatoon, Saskatchewan, Canada

Elan Paluck, MSc, PhD
   Research and Performance Support, Regina Qu'Appelle
   Health Region, Regina, Saskatchewan, Canada

Nancy K. Turner, MSc
   Royal Holloway, University of London, London,
   United Kingdom

Jaime Williams, MA
   Department of Psychology, University of Regina,
   Regina, Saskatchewan, Canada

Introduction

The self-help program that is discussed in this book was developed by pain researchers and health care professionals. This manual was written to address the needs and concerns of older adults who experience chronic pain. Although other books on self-management strategies for chronic pain exist, there are very few materials of this nature for older adults. We believe that a book that is tailored to the needs of older persons makes an important contribution.

North America's population has been changing over the last century, with more and more people now living past age 65. In the year 1900, only about 4% of the population were persons over 65 years of age. According to the United States Census Bureau, close to 13% of the U.S. population is now at least 65 years old, and in approximately 30 years this percentage will have risen to over 20%.

Pain represents one of the most common and universal types of human suffering. It contributes to dramatic reductions in quality of life. Most health conditions that are frequent among older adults carry a substantial burden of pain. According to the *Core Curriculum for Professional Education in Pain*, an important publication of the International Association for the Study of Pain, persistent or chronic pain affects more than 50% of older persons living in the community and more than 80% of those who live in nursing homes.

Often, pain is poorly assessed and treated among older adults, resulting in a great deal of unnecessary physical and emotional suffering. By developing a book specifically for older persons, we are emphasizing that it is possible to avoid having pain in old age and that older adults who have chronic pain can use various strategies to control their pain.

This book includes information about pain-related topics and easy-to-follow techniques and strategies that show you how to better manage your pain. The program is comprehensive and examines many areas of daily life that have a bearing on chronic pain. While developing this book we worked with many seniors and tried to ensure that the information was tailored to their needs. We also took the unique life circumstances of older adults into account.

We recognize that seniors often cope with many health concerns. The pain conditions that older adults have (e.g., osteoarthritis) tend to be different from those typically experienced by younger persons. Moreover, seniors' day-to-day stressors are likely to be different (e.g., lifestyle changes that accompany retirement, *empty nest syndrome,* widowhood). Ideal medication dosages and physical exercise programs are also likely to be different for older persons (e.g., due to sometimes increased general frailty and age-related changes in metabolism). Our book is specifically tailored to address the unique needs of seniors, thus helping fill a gap in the self-help literature. This having been said, several of the techniques that we describe (e.g., procedures designed to improve mood) have been found to be helpful for many pain patients, regardless of age.

Pain is a complex experience that involves mental, physical, and emotional dimensions. Ideally, treatment programs should address the multi-dimensional nature of pain. In fact, programs that focus on a single aspect of pain management (e.g., treating pain with medications alone) are less likely to be successful, especially in the long run. In contrast, treatment programs for pain that are more comprehensive (e.g., do not focus exclusively on medications but include physical therapy and address the psychological consequences of pain) are more likely to succeed. In this book we discuss a wide range of strategies for dealing with pain. We begin by discussing areas that are often overlooked in managing pain, such as relaxation strategies, improving mood, and garnering social support. We then turn to discussion of exercise, modifying the home environment, nutrition, and sleep. In the final chapters, we discuss the development of a collaborative relationship with your physician and provide information about medications. Material for caregivers of older adults who have dementia has also been included in this book. The techniques that are discussed in the various chapters are based on research that has been published by scientists over many years, are designed to address chronic pain, and can contribute to healthy aging.

We suggest that you spend approximately one week on each chapter, completing the book over a 10-week period. This will allow you to learn at a comfortable pace. This book contains a large amount of information and offers many techniques and strategies that could help you to better manage your pain. If you move too quickly, you may experience *information overload.* If this happens, we recommend that you move through the book at a slower pace.

Don't take on too much too soon or try to make too many changes all at the same time. While it is understandable that you want to relieve pain quickly, trying to do too much may lead to confusion and feelings of being overwhelmed. You are advised to follow the content and pace of the book as it unfolds. It's like the tortoise and the hare: slow and steady wins the race!

Overall, the material has been organized and summarized in a way that makes it easy to understand. Within each chapter, there are individual activities that are designed to help you learn and remember the information. There is space for you to write down relevant information as you read about the topics. This way, you can tailor the topics to your own specific needs and concerns.

To receive the most benefit from this program, it is important to be actively involved. Being actively involved will require commitment, time, and effort. For example, many of the techniques that are outlined in this pain management program require practice to learn and master. This will require you to do some *homework.* Only spending one hour a week (or less) engaged in pain management will probably not be enough to have a significant impact on the course of your chronic pain.

Because pain has several components, you may find it helpful to consult with a variety of health professionals about your pain (e.g., your physician, a physical therapist, a dietician) as you complete this book. In fact, we recommend that this manual be used in consultation with appropriate health professionals. It is not meant to be a substitute for professional advice. In Chapter 6 in particular, some physical exercises are discussed. You should not, under any circumstances, attempt these exercises without clearance from a medical practitioner.

As the pain management program progresses, you may not understand certain things right away. That's perfectly normal! No one is expected to perfectly understand all of the material right away. Take your time, review the material, and ask your health professional if you have any questions.

There is evidence that shows that participating in a pain management program can reduce pain and its interference with activities, lead to fewer physician visits, and lessen depression and anxiety. By actively participating in this pain management program, you may experience similar health outcomes and learn how to better manage your pain. At the end of this book, we have included contact information for a variety of organizations that provide seniors with pain management resources in several countries. We hope this information will be helpful to you. We have used the approaches described in this book with many seniors and have special memories of the many successes they have shared with us.

Thomas Hadjistavropoulos

Heather D. Hadjistavropoulos

Disclaimer

The information provided and opinions expressed in this book do not necessarily reflect those of IASP, the publisher of this book. IASP has not verified any of the findings, conclusions, or opinions expressed in this book.

The information in this book is provided for educational purposes and is not intended to be a substitute for professional advice. Because of the rapid advances in the medical sciences and the unique nature of every individual and his or her medical condition, the authors, editors, and publisher recommend independent verification of all information contained herein, including diagnoses and drug dosages. We also strongly recommend that any person embarking on any new program of physical activity (or any other program or activity related to pain assessment and management or to mood management) obtain clearance from a physician and/or other qualified health professional. The authors, editors, and publisher specifically disclaim all responsibility for any liability, loss, injury, risk and/or damage, personal or otherwise, that is incurred as a consequence, directly or indirectly, of the use and application of any of the contents of this book or from any use of any methods, products, instructions, or ideas contained in the material herein.

The persons depicted in the vignettes (which appear in some chapters) do not depict or correspond to any actual person or persons, and all names are fictitious. These vignettes are used for illustrative purposes only.

Acknowledgments

We acknowledge the generous support of our research from the Canadian Institutes of Health Research (CIHR) and from the RBC Foundation. The preparation of this manual took place within the context of a New Emerging Team program funded by CIHR. We are also grateful for all the help and advice of many colleagues and graduate students.

Thomas Hadjistavropoulos

Heather D. Hadjistavropoulos

RONALD R. MARTIN, PHD, RD PSYCH.
THOMAS HADJISTAVROPOULOS, PHD, RD PSYCH.
HEATHER D. HADJISTAVROPOULOS, PHD, RD PSYCH.

CHAPTER ONE

Pain among Seniors

Stan

Stan is not sure exactly when it happened, but over time he developed a very bad limp. Because he was compensating for his bad leg, his back also began to hurt. He looked upon people who could walk normally with great envy—including people much older than he was. He said to himself, "I'm old before my time."

Stan talked to his family doctor about the pain. The doctor said it was "just part of getting older." It depressed Stan to think about it, but within a year or two after the onset of his leg pain, his life had become very different.

On the golf course, Stan could no longer swing the club around completely. Walking left him hurting, even with the help of a cane. Shopping caused his leg pain to flare up to the point that he could not even participate in normal conversation. Each step was painful. Slowing down, speeding up, stopping and starting, stepping off curbs and uneven surfaces also caused him pain. Because every second step resulted in a sharp stab of pain, he grew quiet and appeared not to be interested in others.

Simple things such as rising out of a chair after dinner required a great deal of mental effort. A few minutes before he actually stood up, he would start bracing himself for the surge of pain he knew he would experience. Pain was controlling his life, and he felt he couldn't do a thing about it.

1

Have you ever been told that you had better learn to live with pain because it is normal for older adults? As it turns out, this is one of many myths about seniors that contributes to undertreatment of pain in this age group. Stan's situation is not uncommon. Fortunately, there are things that can be done to help you manage pain, increase your enjoyment of life, and improve your mood.

This chapter describes the frequency of pain among older adults and the common diseases and medical problems that cause pain. We will also highlight various other myths about pain among seniors and will help you develop a personal understanding of how chronic pain can affect your life. Finally, in this chapter, we will review some of the benefits people experience when their pain is properly treated.

How Common is Pain among Older Adults?

Pain is a very common concern among older adults. Persistent pain is the primary symptom of many common chronic diseases of aging. Researchers Andrew Cook and Michael Thomas reported that 50% of older adults experience pain on a daily basis, and another 28% experience it at least once a week. In another study of seniors living in the community, Paula Mobily and her colleagues found that 86% experienced significant pain in the year prior to their participation in the study, with close to 60% having multiple pain complaints. In the United States, estimates from the National Council on Aging indicate that pain is twice as common among those aged 60 years and over than in those under age 60.

Common Pain Problems

An initial step toward managing your pain more effectively involves gaining knowledge about pain. To start off, it may be helpful to take a moment to review some common health problems that involve pain. According to a Statistics Canada report, the following is a list of chronic health problems that typically involve pain. The list includes the estimated percentage of seniors who experience each of these problems.

Disease or Health Problem	Percentage of Seniors Affected
Arthritis/rheumatism	40%
Back problems (not including arthritis)	18%
Heart disease	17%
Diabetes	11%
Chronic bronchitis/emphysema	6%
Stomach/intestinal ulcers	5%
Migraine	4%

Do you experience any of these health problems? If not, do you know other seniors who do? The answer is probably "yes!" The widespread occurrence of these medical problems helps us understand why pain is such a common experience among older adults.

Inadequate Management of Pain among Older Adults

A recent survey of members of the American Pain Society, organized by Dr. Betty Ferrell and her colleagues, found that one of the most pressing ethical issues for health care providers concerned the under-management of pain among seniors. Moreover, a 2001 Canadian Senate Standing Committee Report and a Health Canada document raised serious concerns about pain management in later life and about the quality of care available to many older adults who are terminally ill. You may be wondering why pain is undertreated in seniors. There are several possible explanations.

Seniors often do not report the full extent of their pain. Many older adults may be reluctant to report pain to their doctors. Seniors sometimes believe that pain must be endured and that, if they report it, they may be seen as nuisances or complainers. Also, they may believe in the traditional doctor-patient relationship in which the doctor leads and the patient follows. Seniors who have these traditional relationships may assume that their physicians will ask about pain.

As a result, these seniors often don't mention pain during office visits. Older patients may also have sensory impairments—hearing difficulties, for instance—that interfere with effective communication. They may feel nervous or embarrassed when talking to their doctors about certain medical problems, including pain.

Health care professionals may not always assess pain properly. Some older adults may require more time to describe their pain symptoms and relevant medical histories. However, due to changes in the health-care system, doctors have less time to spend with patients. Pain may be pushed to the side while other medical problems are given higher priority. The hectic pace of the doctor's schedule, along with the busy and chaotic atmospheres of many doctors' offices, may leave the health care professional with little time to ask specifically about pain. Furthermore, many health care providers do not have easy access to pain assessment tools (such as systematic questionnaires) that are appropriate for seniors.

Myths about Pain in Seniors

Seniors and even some health professionals may believe certain myths about aging and pain that undermine effective pain management. You may be surprised to find that some common beliefs about pain in seniors are based on inaccurate information. Dispelling myths about pain assessment and management will help you become better informed and better prepared to manage your pain.

The following are examples of common myths about pain. Use Section 3 of the checklist at the end of this chapter (page 9) to detemine whether you hold any beliefs that are considered to be myths about pain in old age. Then read the section below to learn the reasons why these views are considered myths.

Myth: Experiencing pain is a natural part of growing old.

Fact: Although pain accompanies many illnesses that affect older people (such as osteoarthritis or cancer), it is not the result of old age, but a consequence of disease, illness, or injury that needs to be treated or managed. If we think of pain as a natural part of being old, we may be less inclined to treat it effectively. Persistent pain needs to be managed regardless of a person's age.

4

Myth: Older adults suffer less than younger persons when they have pain problems.

Fact: Older adults are likely to be affected by pain at least as much as younger persons.

Myth: "I don't have the right to ask questions about my pain."

Fact: As a patient, you have every right to information regarding your pain and its proper treatment. You can discuss various treatment options with your physician.

Myth: Older adults can't tolerate strong painkillers.

Fact: Opioid (narcotic) painkillers, such as morphine, codeine, and oxycodone, can be very appropriate medications depending on an older person's condition. The selection and dose of the painkiller are very important since some are better tolerated than others. If these medications are appropriate for you, your doctor may start at a low dose and increase it slowly in order to avoid side effects. There is no definitive or specific dose for these painkillers. According to an American Geriatrics Society panel, which developed guidelines for the management of pain in older persons, the best dose is the one that gives the most effective relief with the lowest number of side effects. Discuss these issues with your doctor.

Myth: Analgesic pills (painkillers) are the only means of treating pain.

Fact: Although analgesic medication is often a first step in controlling pain, it need not be your only line of defense. Alternative or complementary approaches to pain management can help provide effective relief. For example, physical therapy, psychological coping strategies, massages, hot and cold packs, and relaxation techniques may all help you manage your pain, increase your physical functioning, relieve stress, and improve your quality of life.

5

Myth: "Aside from taking my medications or using alternative approaches to pain management, there's nothing I can do to control my pain."

Fact: In addition to medications and alternative pain management approaches, you can also incorporate simple activities into your day to help control and cope with your pain. These include acknowledging your feelings about how pain affects you, getting adequate rest, eating a variety of healthy foods, and engaging in regular forms of medically approved exercise.

Myth: "I don't have to describe my pain to my doctor. He or she will know all about it."

Fact: You are the only person who knows how your pain feels and how severe it is, so it is very important to tell your doctor about it. Your doctor, in turn, must listen to, acknowledge, and have confidence in your account and help you to do something about your pain.

Consequences of Chronic Pain

If you, or others you know, suffer from chronic pain, you are probably familiar with the consequences. The impact of pain is most obvious in the physical sense. Pain involves physical suffering. However, pain also affects many other areas of life that may not be immediately obvious, including social, emotional, and mental well-being.

 Remember Stan from the beginning of this chapter? His pain caused him to become less active and affected his relationships, his energy, and his mood.

Consider some of the many ways in which pain may be affecting your life, and record these in the checklist at the end of this chapter. The examples below represent areas that can change with effective pain treatment, including self-management. It is important to remember that pain can:

- Make you less active and interfere with your ability to do things such as walking, bending, or lifting

- Limit your ability to carry out routine daily activities such as cooking, cleaning, and even bathing

- Make it hard to get to sleep, or stay asleep

- Interfere with your relationships and activities with your spouse, as well as your children, grandchildren, and friends

- Limit your activities and lead to increased loneliness and isolation

- Change your appetite by making you want to eat more or not at all

- Drain your energy, leaving you fatigued

- Limit your ability to concentrate

- Increase your feelings of anxiety and helplessness

- Make you feel irritable, depressed, and downhearted

Benefits of Pain Self-Management

As we've discussed earlier, chronic pain is common among older adults. There are also many possible sources of pain. Keep in mind, however, that it is possible to take an active role in managing your pain more effectively. In the chapters ahead, we'll show you how to begin to take control of your pain problem. When pain is well managed, older adults may be spared a great deal of physical suffering. In addition, seniors can expect a number of other advantages. In the checklist at the end of this chapter, record the benefits you hope to achieve. The following are examples of goals that many of our patients have set.

- Have more energy

- Improve my activity and movement

- Achieve greater independence (be able to shop, cook, or perform household tasks)

- Feel more "in charge" of my life

- ⊚ Have better sleep

- ⊚ Improve my appetite

- ⊚ Develop more satisfying relationships (spend more "pain-free" time with others)

- ⊚ Increase my concentration

- ⊚ Improve my mood (feel happier and more positive)

- ⊚ Improve my communication with health care providers

 Stan followed the exercises described in this book. He used relaxation techniques, identified and changed his negative thoughts, asked for support, and changed his exercises and medications. Within a very short period of time, he improved his level of activity, found new activities that he enjoyed, and improved both his mood and his relationships with his family.

Summary

The purpose of this chapter was to provide information about chronic pain among older adults and review some myths about pain in old age. Clearly, ongoing pain is common among seniors. However, the exact nature of chronic pain is not the same for everyone. You might say that no two seniors will experience a chronic pain condition in exactly the same way. For this reason, it is important for you to consider how the information in this chapter applies specifically to you.

Use the questions in the checklist to review whether you have any of the common conditions associated with pain. Which myths about chronic pain among seniors do you or others you know hold? In what ways has pain affected your life? Gaining a better understanding of the nature of chronic pain, and its effects on your life, will provide you with a solid background for discussions that lay ahead in this book. In those discussions, we will aim to help you achieve some of the benefits we have described in this chapter.

Pain Checklist

1. **Which health care conditions do you have that are commonly associated with pain?**

   ○ Arthritis/rheumatism   ○ Back problems   ○ Heart disease

   ○ Diabetes   ○ Chronic bronchitis   ○ Emphysema

   ○ Migraine   ○ Other _____

   ○ Stomach/intestinal ulcers

2. **How often do you experience pain?**

   ○ Daily   ○ Every 2 to 3 days   ○ Once a week

   ○ Every other week   ○ Once a month   ○ Less often

3. **Do you believe any of the myths below?**

   ○ Experiencing pain is a natural part of growing old.

   ○ Older adults suffer less than younger persons when they have a pain problem.

   ○ The only way to treat pain is with analgesic pills (painkillers).

   ○ Aside from taking my pain medications or using alternative approaches to pain management, there's nothing I can do to control my pain.

   ○ I don't have the right to ask questions about my pain.

   ○ I don't have to describe my pain to my doctor. He or she will know about my pain.

   Read the chapter to learn why these myths are not true.

4. **Have you noticed that you are less able to do the things you want to do because of pain? Check those that apply to you.**

   My pain

   ○ forces me to be less active, interfering with walking, bending, and lifting.

Chapter One | *Pain among Seniors*

Pain Checklist continued...

○ limits my ability to carry out routine daily activities such as cooking, cleaning, and bathing.

○ interrupts my sleep, either making it difficult for me to get to sleep or to stay asleep.

○ interferes with my relationships, by making me cancel or avoid activities with children, grandchildren, and friends.

○ has changed my appetite, making me want to either eat more or eat less.

○ drains my energy, leaving me fatigued, even when I've had enough time to rest.

○ limits my ability to concentrate on things like reading or watching television.

○ makes me anxious and tense.

○ makes me feel sad, depressed, or helpless.

○ makes me irritable.

_____ Add up the number of check marks in this section. The higher your score out of 10, the greater impact your pain is having on you. Can you think of other ways in which pain has had a negative impact on your life? If so, write your thoughts in the spaces below.

_____

_____

_____

_____

_____

Pain Checklist continued...

5. **Note the changes you would like to see as a result of following this manual.**

   ○ More energy

   ○ Improved movement

   ○ Improved activity

   ○ Greater independence (be able to go shopping, cook, do homemaking chores)

   ○ Feeling more "in charge" of my life

   ○ Improved sleep

   ○ More satisfying relationships (be able to spend more *"pain-free"* time with others)

   ○ Better concentration

   ○ Improved mood (feel happier and more positive)

   ○ Better communication with health care providers

At the end of this book, we'll ask you to review the list again. By then, we hope that you will see for yourself that following the strategies we outline in these pages can have a significant impact on your life.

RONALD R. MARTIN, PHD, RD PSYCH.
THOMAS HADJISTAVROPOULOS, PHD, RD PSYCH.
JAIME WILLIAMS, MA
HEATHER D. HADJISTAVROPOULOS, PHD, RD PSYCH.

CHAPTER TWO

Pain and Psychology

Evelyn

Evelyn was a driven person. During her career as an office manager, she worked at a relentless pace that earned her promotions. However, a few years after she retired, she began to experience chronic pain in her upper back. On several occasions, she went to her doctor for help, but when she was asked to describe her pain, she couldn't express the details and became flustered.

She resigned herself to accepting her pain because she believed that she couldn't control it no matter what she did. So when she worked on projects around the house, she would push herself until the pain was so great that she was forced to stop. When asked why she pushed herself so hard, she would say, "I might as well get as much work done as I can while I'm not in pain." Whenever she overdid it, she was forced to stop all of her projects and recuperate for a day or two while taking extra pain medication.

After feeling that she was at the mercy of her pain for years, Evelyn started to become depressed. One day a friend asked her why she seemed so blue. Evelyn responded, "It's impossible to feel happy when you're dealing with back pain like mine."

Understanding Pain

Sometimes, health care professionals suggest that their patients with chronic pain visit a psychologist. When this happens, patients may worry that they are being told that the pain is *in their heads*. Many people mistakenly think of pain as a purely physical sensation. However, pain involves both physical and psychological reactions. The International Association for the Study of Pain (IASP), the largest and most prestigious group of pain researchers and clinicians in the world, defines pain as a physical sensation that involves negative emotions. Pain (especially chronic pain) is often accompanied by strong emotions including worry, fear, frustration, anger, disgust, and sadness. In addition, pain can lead to chronic negative emotional states such as depression.

Health psychologists (psychologists who work in the management and prevention of medical illness) can help people change the way they think about their pain (which is discussed in detail in later chapters) and the way they react to it. They also show people how to manage negative feelings associated with pain (such as depression, anxiety, and even sleep problems) and to avoid the negative psychological consequences of pain. In fact, psychological pain management programs have been shown to reduce levels of pain, improve mood, decrease health care costs, and improve quality of life. To find a psychologist specializing in work with pain patients, contact your state, provincial, or national psychological association.

Negative Emotions

Negative emotions that accompany pain may include:

- **Fear:** *an unpleasant feeling of risk or danger.*

- **Anxiety:** *a feeling of unease or worry accompanied by physical symptoms such as rapid heart beat, faintness, and trembling.*

- **Sadness:** *a state of gloominess.*

- **Depression:** *persistent sadness that often involves a loss of interest in activities, feelings of pessimism, and other related difficulties.*

- **Disgust:** *strong feelings of dislike.*

- ◎ **Frustration:** *a sense of discomfort and disappointment when a person cannot achieve certain goals.*

- ◎ **Anger:** *a strong emotion that often results from the feeling that one has been wronged.*

- ◎ **Irritability:** *feeling cranky and sensitive.*

- ◎ **Worthlessness:** *a feeling that one lacks value.*

- ◎ **Boredom:** *a lack of interest in activities or feeling empty inside.*

Pain Diary

The first step in taking control of your pain is to understand it. If you learn how to monitor your pain, you will be in a much better position to try different management techniques and to find out which ones work best for you.

In order to monitor your pain, we strongly recommend that you complete a pain diary. There are many reasons why this is important. You can us e the pain diary to track pain over time, which will help you to identify the specific situations that make your pain better or worse.

If you gain a better understanding of the things that happen before your pain starts or worsens, you will be able to change your behavior and may lessen your pain or even avoid it altogether. To do so, it may be useful to examine the thoughts, feelings, behaviors, people, and situations that tend to cause or worsen your pain.

- ◎ **Thoughts:** *self-defeating thoughts about yourself or your pain.*

- ◎ **Feelings:** *intense or lingering feelings (usually negative).*

- ◎ **Behaviors:** *taking part in activities that put stress on weakened parts of the body for too long without rest periods. Remaining inactive for extended periods of time.*

- ◎ **People:** *spending time with people who tend to upset you or who constantly focus on pain.*

- ◎ **Places:** *visiting places that may be associated with increased stress and agitation. Stress and pain can also be related to lighting, noise, or the pace of activity.*

15

Patients tell us that they are surprised to find triggers they were not aware of before using a pain diary. Armed with such knowledge, you can learn to control your pain by changing the things that make it worse. You can also bring the diary to appointments with your doctor to help you describe your pain.

Researchers have found that keeping a diary is invaluable when people are trying to make beneficial changes in their lives. Diaries are much more important than most people realize because they help us "stay on track" when we are trying to effect changes in our lives such as making better nutritional choices, improving sleep habits, or giving up cigarettes.

 As you can see from the sample diary on the next page, Evelyn rated the severity of her pain on a daily basis, noting when pain was at its worst and to what degree it interfered with her activities and mood. On the form, she also noted which pain management strategies she used. This helped her systematically keep track of how her pain and mood were affected by the strategies she was using.

A pain diary sheet is included at the end of this chapter. Feel free to make copies for your personal use.

Summary

Now that you have read this chapter, you are in a better position to see the connections between chronic pain and psychological reactions such as sadness and disappointment. Specifically, you might recognize that negative emotions (e.g., depression, anxiety, anger) are linked to chronic pain.

This chapter has also given you ideas about how to monitor your pain. You will find this particularly helpful as you begin to implement the strategies described in upcoming chapters.

Evelyn's Diary

1. **Put a box around the number that shows the lowest your pain was today. Circle the number that shows your average level of pain today. Make a triangle around the number that shows how severe your pain was today.**

    0   1   2   [3]   4   5   (6)   7   △8   9   10

    no pain   *moderate pain*   *severe pain*

2. **When was your pain at its worst today? (check all that apply)**

    ✓ morning   ___ afternoon   ✓ evening   ___ during the night

3. **What words would you use to describe your pain today?**

    ✓ throbbing   ___ shooting   ___ stabbing   ✓ sharp

    ___ cramping   ___ gnawing   ___ burning   ✓ aching

    ___ heavy   ___ tender   ✓ splitting   ___ tiring

    ___ sickening   ___ fearful   ___ punishing

4. **Rate the degree to which your pain interfered with your ability to carry out important daily activities today?**

    0   1   2   3   4   5   6   7   (8)   9   10

    not at all   *moderate impact*   *severe impact*

5. **Which activities were most difficult for you today?**

    Walking, sitting, housecleaning.

6. **What words would you use to describe your emotions today? (e.g., sad, happy, irritable, tired, energized, frustrated, disinterested, engaged, content, bored, patient)**

    Sad, irritable, tired.

    Continued...

Evelyn's Diary continued...

7. **What made your pain worse today? Were any negative thoughts, feelings, behaviors, people, or places linked to your pain?**

   Sitting around in the crowded mall feeling sad and thinking about how I'd like to be out doing other things. Doing household chores.

8. **What made your pain better today?**

   Pacing my activities, relaxing, calling a friend.

Daily Pain Diary

Make copies of this diary and complete it on a daily basis. Filling out the diary is quick and easy, and you don't have to rely on your memory for details regarding your pain.

Date: _____

1. **Put a box around the number that shows the lowest your pain was today. Circle the number that shows your average level of pain today. Make a triangle around the number that shows how severe your pain was today.**

0	1	2	3	4	5	6	7	8	9	10
no pain					*moderate pain*				*severe pain*	

2. **When was your pain at its worst today?** *(check all that apply)*

   ___ morning   ___ afternoon   ___ evening   ___ during the night

3. **What words would you use to describe your pain today?**

   ___ throbbing   ___ shooting   ___ stabbing   ___ sharp

   ___ cramping   ___ gnawing   ___ burning   ___ aching

   ___ heavy   ___ tender   ___ splitting   ___ tiring

   ___ sickening   ___ fearful   ___ punishing

4. **Rate the degree to which your pain interfered with your ability to carry out important daily activities today.**

0	1	2	3	4	5	6	7	8	9	10
not at all					*moderate impact*				*severe impact*	

   Continued...

Daily Pain Diary continued...

5. **Which activities were most difficult for you today?**

_____

_____

6. **What words would you use to describe your emotions today?**
   (e.g., sad, happy, irritable, tired, energized, frustrated,
   disinterested, engaged, content, bored, patient)

_____

_____

7. **What made your pain worse today? Were any negative**
   thoughts, feelings, behaviors, people, or places linked to
   your pain?

_____

_____

8. **What made your pain better today?**

_____

_____

In this book we are recommending techniques
that can help you overcome negative emotions
that are linked to pain.

RONALD R. MARTIN, PHD, RD PSYCH.
THOMAS HADJISTAVROPOULOS, PHD, RD PSYCH.
HEATHER D. HADJISTAVROPOULOS, PHD, RD PSYCH.
SANDRA M. LEFORT, RN, PHD
SHANNON FUCHS-LACELLE, PHD

CHAPTER THREE

Taking Control:
Effective Pain Management

Louise

While standing on a chair to reach an item on a top shelf, Louise lost her balance and fell. Miraculously, she didn't injure her hips or her knees. However, she did break her arm and injure her shoulder. The doctor explained that her bones were some-what brittle because of her osteoporosis.

Louise experienced pain for a time as her arm and shoulder mended. She focused on the pain, noticing different sensations, and was worried about not making a full recovery. She was an active volunteer in her community, so having an arm in a cast was a serious setback.

Over time, the doctors realized that her arm was not mending properly. Medical complications prolonged the healing process and worsened her pain. Louise focused on her pain almost constantly. She thought she would never be able to return to her previous volunteer duties at her local Red Cross. Gradually she found that when she spent her days thinking about the pain in her arm and shoulder, she became steadily more depressed and irritable. Her family and friends noticed the change in her mood. They expressed their concern that she was thinking too much about her arm and that this did not seem to be helping it heal.

Some people, like Louise, feel helpless when dealing with pain. They think that pain is something that can either be treated by a doctor or must simply be lived with. Misconceptions such as these often make people feel helpless, that there is little that they can do to manage pain. In this chapter, we will help you find strategies to take active control of your pain. The psychosocial pain management procedures described in this chapter have helped thousands of patients control their pain. More specifically, this chapter will help you (a) learn ways to distract yourself from pain; (b) learn more effective techniques for achieving a state of relaxation, which can help with pain management; and (c) learn to balance activity and relaxation through pacing (breaking down activities and projects into small, manageable chunks). We will also consider different ways of thinking about pain and about one's daily life.

Distraction

Most people tend to pay a great deal of attention to their pain. Physical suffering definitely gets your attention! However, when people with chronic pain spend too much time focusing on their pain, strong negative emotions tend to become frequent.

The presence of pain includes the following: (1) attention to pain and (2) a negative emotional reaction (e.g., sadness or anger). So, if a person with a chronic pain condition (e.g., arthritis) shifts his or her attention away from suffering by laughing at a funny movie, is that person technically *in pain* at that moment? A physical sensation is still present. However, if the person is not aware of the sensation and the pain is not accompanied by a negative emotional reaction, the suffering can diminish quite dramatically.

Distraction is often used in pain management. Many dentists employ this technique by equipping their offices with televisions that patients can watch during dental procedures. An interesting television program makes a painful experience more tolerable. Distraction involves directing your attention away from pain and focusing on something else such as a conversation with a friend, music, a hobby, or a television program.

It may not be possible to use distraction at all times. There are probably periods during your day, however, when focusing on something else may help you improve your mood and forget about your pain.

 Louise realized that her family and friends had a point: she was thinking too much about her painful arm and shoulder. So she decided to do something about it by learning to use distraction to manage her pain. One day, she rented the movie "Grumpy Old Men" starring Jack Lemmon and Walter Matthau. She couldn't stop laughing. When the movie was over, she was amazed that she had hardly been aware of the pain in her arm and shoulder for almost two hours! She was pleasantly surprised and relieved that she had found a way to manage her pain and improve her mood, even if it was only for a short time. It gave her a much-desired break.

Relaxation

You may wonder what relaxation has to do with pain. According to the National Institutes of Health Technology Assessment Panel on Integration of Behavioral and Relaxation Approaches, research and clinical practice have shown that the use of relaxation techniques can reduce pain, anxiety, and stress and can also lead to better sleep. This is especially true for muscle pain (such as most kinds of low back pain) and headaches. Tension aggravates muscle pain and headaches. Relaxation helps loosen your tense muscles and can help relieve your pain.

Even if you are certain that relaxation will help you manage your pain more effectively, you might think that you already know how to relax. We urge you to take the time to read the following section on relaxation techniques even if you have practiced relaxation in the past. In this chapter we describe several different techniques to give you more options for achieving a relaxed state. Many people are surprised by the effectiveness of these techniques when they use them on a regular basis.

Diaphragmatic (Belly) Breathing

In many cases, people breathe by taking shallow breaths into the chest while holding in the stomach. This type of breathing is especially common in stressful situations and is called *chest breathing.* One problem is that chest breathing makes use of muscles in the upper chest, neck, and shoulders. If you experience chronic pain in these areas, chest breathing may tend to worsen your pain. In addition, since chest breathing is associated with tension, it may also lead to increased feelings of anxiety when you are experiencing stress.

Diaphragmatic breathing involves sending your breath down into your belly. Breathing this way makes more use of your diaphragm (an important muscle located at the base of your lungs). By concentrating on using your diaphragm while breathing, you place less strain on the muscles in your upper chest, neck, and shoulders. This type of breathing may help reduce your feelings of anxiety and at the same time give you a sense of control over your pain.

Babies engage in diaphragmatic breathing naturally. Watch how a baby breathes and you can see for yourself! Unfortunately, as many people age, they gradually shift toward chest breathing. Therefore, relearning to breathe from the diaphragm takes some effort.

We recommend using the following procedure at least twice a day.

Mastering this form of relaxation can take a little time. Try practicing this exercise for 10 minutes each time. Once you become familiar with the technique, you can use it more frequently and in different settings. You will also find that you will be better able to deal with distractions and focus your attention on achieving a state of relaxation more quickly.

1. Start by choosing a quiet environment where you will not be interrupted. Sit in a comfortable position. Pick a chair that has good back support and allows you to sit up straight. Arm rests and head support are also important.

2. Close your eyes and remain passive and relaxed.

3. While keeping an upright posture, place one hand on your stomach and the other on your chest.

4. Take approximately three seconds to breathe in and three seconds to breathe out. As you breathe, notice which of your hands moves the most. When resting, the hand on your stomach should have the most movement. If you are a chest breather, the hand on your chest will move more than the hand on your stomach.

5. Make the hand on your stomach move out as you breathe in. Try to make sure that the hand on your chest moves much less. This will take some effort and practice. Another way to practice this exercise is to lie down on a flat surface and position your hands the same way. You can place a pillow under your knees to make yourself more comfortable and take the strain off your lower back.

6. Some of our patients have difficulty getting the knack of breathing with the belly because they are so used to shallow chest breathing. If this happens to you, you may want to try the same hand positions when lying in bed at night. Chances are that just before falling asleep you will begin to belly breathe. Focusing on belly breathing just before falling asleep will help you reproduce it at other times.

 When Louise tried the belly breathing technique, she found she was breathing mostly with her chest. This chest breathing style made her pain worse, and it certainly didn't do much to reduce her feelings of anxiety and discomfort!

Word Enhancement

The Relaxation Response is a classic book written by Dr. Herbert Benson of Harvard University. During certain relaxation exercises, Dr. Benson recommends that you repeat certain words to yourself as you inhale and exhale. You could, for example, count *one* when you inhale and *two* when you exhale. Another possibility is to say "one" when you inhale and "relax" when you exhale. Focusing on these words, rather than on outside distractions, will allow feelings of relaxation to emerge.

When you first begin using this technique, you might have trouble dealing with distractions such as noises in your immediate environment or thoughts that keep jumping into your mind. If this happens, use the distraction as an indicator that you need to refocus your attention on your words (e.g., *one — relax*). With regular practice, even the most anxious people can learn to relax effectively and to use this procedure to help manage pain more effectively.

 As part of her breathing exercise, Louise used the words "breathe in" as she inhaled and "relax" as she exhaled.

Imagery

Have you ever used your imagination to form a mental picture of a pleasant setting, or to *play a movie* of a fond memory in your mind? If so, what effect did this have on your thoughts, feelings, and bodily sensations? It is probably safe to assume that, in most cases, you probably experienced positive thoughts, felt more relaxed and happy, and became less aware of any physical discomfort. The ability to use visual imagery (mental scenes) can help you to relax as well as to manage your pain.

Many people think of pain as something that infiltrates the body. People may provide a visual description of their pain as a *hot poker* or as if an animal were chewing on a particular body part. However, imagining pain in this way leads to greater disability. In other words, if you imagine your pain as a metal poker in your back, you are much more likely to feel down and perhaps to limit your daily activities. Research has shown that imagining pain in other ways allows people to feel more energized and able to do the things they enjoy.

Visualization may be used to counter the negative images of pain and suffering. For example, if asked to describe what your pain feels like, you might say, *It feels like my back is on fire*. By using imagery, you can imagine taking a bucket of ice water and dousing your pain until it turns from fiery red to blue. As you are imagining this, you may possibly feel the pain becoming cool. Alternatively, you might visualize a hot water bottle warming and soothing your muscles. As you imagine this feeling, it is possible that you might actually experience the warmth and relief that a hot water bottle might provide.

A number of imagery exercises are described below. Try them and discover which exercises bring you the greatest relief. When using imagery,

26

try to use all of your senses: think of what the image looks like, what it sounds, smells, and feels like. The more senses you use in imagery the more vivid and effective the image will be. Before you try the exercises, prepare yourself by doing the following:

1. Sit in a comfortable position, preferably in a chair with arms. Keep your arms and legs uncrossed.

2. Close your eyes.

3. Use your diaphragmatic (belly) breathing technique.

4. Begin to think about an image:

    Beach. Imagine lying on a beach. You hear the waves crashing against the shore and the sound of the sea birds. You smell the salty air and feel the warmth of the sun on your skin. Your muscles feel warm and relaxed. You feel at peace. You notice some discomfort in your back. You realize that the stones from the beach are pressing against your back. It does not hurt but is slightly uncomfortable. As you watch the waves, you forget about the stones that you are lying on and instead focus on the warmth and sunshine.

    Cottage. You are spending the night at your cottage in the woods. You light a fire and lie down in your bed nearby. You can hear the crackling of the wood and smell the sweet smoke. The warmth fills your entire body. You feel heavy and sink deeper and deeper into the bed. You see your pain float out of your body into the air. You feel your discomfort drift away. It mingles with the smoke in the fireplace and disappears up the chimney.

5. Once you have tried the images, feel free to change them to your liking, keeping in mind that the goal is to use imagery in such a way as to improve your well-being and reduce the pain.

Louise sometimes imagined her pain as a red hot poker stabbing her in the shoulder. Focusing on such negative images made her pain worse. After she learned about relaxation, she used the cottage image with the warmth of the fire relaxing her body. At other times, she imagined a waterfall running down her shoulder and cooling the pain away.

Sometimes, we are not be able to recognize changes when they occur gradually. Use the sheets at the end of this chapter *(Relaxation Questions* and *Relaxation Monitoring Sheet)* to monitor your relaxation practice (pages 34–35). This is important because using the monitoring sheets will make it easier for you to keep track of your progress and see results over time.

Balancing Rest and Activity

Some people who have chronic pain find themselves resting quite a bit. This is understandable. When the pain first appears, resting seems like a good idea. However, over time, resting can become more of a *lifestyle.* When people with chronic pain rest too much and engage in too few activities, they may become out of shape. Dr. Bortz, a retired physician and geriatrician, cautions seniors about the *disuse syndrome.* His advice reflects the old adage *use it or lose it.* Did you know, for instance, that you can lose up to 10% of your muscle strength and muscle mass by being inactive for just one week?

Muscles that are not exercised can *atrophy,* which means that they become tighter, shorter, and weaker. When muscles atrophy, any kind of movement or activity can be uncomfortable (which may be unrelated to the person's chronic pain condition). In addition, people who rest all the time may find that they *get winded* and tire more easily. Dr. Bortz's research suggests that physical inactivity leads to a decline in virtually all bodily functions, including one's mental functioning!

While some people with chronic pain rest too much, others ignore their pain and push themselves to continue with activities. These people frequently rely on extra pain medication to help them get through the day. After periods of high activity, these people often *fall apart* and need time to recover.

Pacing is a technique you can use to balance activity and rest. It requires you to set a *realistic* schedule of activity and rest periods. This schedule will allow you to accomplish your daily goals, while keeping your pain under control.

Older adults with chronic pain vary greatly in terms of how much they can do without bringing on their pain or making it worse. Pacing varies according to both the individual and the activity. For example, seniors with hip problems might adopt a more relaxed pace for walking and a more aggressive pace for lighter or less aerobic activities.

Your own experience will help you to determine the pace that is right for you. For example, you may know that you can work at something comfortably for half an hour before you need to stop and rest for 5 or 10 minutes. However, if you are not sure, one way to determine a good pace is by trial and error. Start off with a conservative approach. This means engaging in the activity for a short interval (e.g., 5 to 10 minutes) followed by a rest period of a few minutes. Adjust your pace according to the pain that you experience. The idea is to determine how long you can do something without pain (or without making your pain worse) and to schedule rest breaks at the right time.

Working to schedule involves scheduling your activities to include a rest break before your pain forces you to stop. Working to tolerance, on the other hand, involves pushing yourself to your limit. This is when pain begins to get worse, and it does not need to happen!

Louise decided to take control of her pain. She started pacing herself by "working to schedule" and taking rest breaks. At first it was difficult to schedule breaks because she felt that she was giving up or walking away from her responsibilities. However, over time, she realized that a short break left her feeling refreshed and able to continue for longer periods of time.

Examine Your Thoughts

Did you know that your thought patterns can affect how you feel? The things you think about, and the beliefs you have about yourself and the world around you, can have an impact on important factors such as mood, self-esteem, and self-confidence. If your thoughts are negative or irrational, problems may arise. For example, if you think, *I'm no good at learning new things. I always end up failing,* you will probably avoid trying new things and feel less confident about yourself and your abilities.

This kind of thought pattern might also result in feelings of depression. If this is the case, it may be necessary to change these problematic thoughts by learning to recognize and evaluate them, then replace them with healthier, adaptive thoughts (i.e., thoughts that are beneficial to you and help you to adjust to your living situation). This process is broadly referred to as *cognitive restructuring.* Cognitive restructuring is a technical term that means identifying negative thinking patterns and replacing them with more adaptive thoughts.

The way you think can have an enormous impact on your pain. For example, if you are convinced that you are stuck with your pain and that it will never get better, you will probably develop a sense of power-lessness. Further, these kinds of thoughts may lead to increased anxiety and muscle tension, which will make the pain worse.

Famous researchers and clinicians such as Aaron Beck, Albert Ellis, and David Burns have identified several different types of thinking that may lead to problems with mood and self-esteem. Here are some examples:

- **Focusing on one negative event and applying it to all other events.**

  Example: I tried going for a walk once and ended up in pain. I'll never be able to walk or do any type of exercise again.

- **Imagining the worst possible consequences in a given situation.**

  Example: If I try any type of exercise I'll probably injure myself somehow and end up in a hospital bed on massive doses of painkillers.

- **Drawing conclusions that are unwarranted based on the facts at hand.**

  Example: Ever since that last solar eclipse my pain has gotten better. I hope the next eclipse comes soon– I could use some more relief.

- **Seeing your pain in "black and white" terms.**

  Example: When it comes to my pain, I'm either functioning just fine or I'm completely incapacitated. There's no in-between for me.

- **Making too much or too little of your pain based on the available facts.** This is known as *magnifying* or *minimizing*.

  Example of magnifying: My doctor frowned when he was examining my bad knee. That must mean my knee is really bad.

  Example of minimizing: I must ignore my pain completely and do all of my physical work without a break.

- **Taking responsibility for something that is unrelated to you.**

  Example: I've had pain for several years now. I must have done something wrong to deserve this suffering.

- **Discounting any positive experiences.**

  Example: Sure, I managed to work for several hours without pain, but that was just luck.

- **Believing that nothing works** (*i.e., no interventions would be helpful*).

  Example: I've tried every treatment there is. Nothing works for me.

The first step in changing problematic thoughts is to become aware of them. If you have trouble remembering whether or not you engage in any of these ways of thinking, you can record your thoughts using the monitoring sheet printed at the end of this chapter.

Challenge Your Thoughts

If you identify a thought such as one of those listed above, try substituting it with a more realistic and adaptive one. Remember, however, that it takes regular work and practice (consistently substituting maladaptive ways of thinking with adaptive ones) before more positive ways of thinking about pain become a natural part of the way that you think. Many people have pain, but some have a better quality of life than others because of the things that they do to gain control of their situation.

Be persistent!

Here are some examples of maladative thoughts and adaptive substitutes:

Instead of thinking, *Stop whining about your pain,* **or** *Don't be a quitter, get the job done first and you can rest later,* **try substituting,** *Pace yourself, you'll get more done and lessen your pain.*

Instead of thinking, *Because I have pain, I can never be happy,* **try substituting,** *Yes, I have pain but there are things that I can do to increase the quality of my life, despite the pain. I can talk to a friend, listen to music or read a book. I can also talk to my doctor about better pain management.*

Behavioral Experiments

Sometimes, you may have difficulty changing certain maladaptive thoughts. In addition to using the techniques described above, you can also test out your thoughts. Psychologists sometimes refer to this as a *behavioral experiment*. For instance, you may have the following thought: *Because I am in pain, I cannot meet and socialize with new people.* You can test this thought by joining a club or a recreational class (perhaps at the local seniors' education center) to see how many people you can get to know. Choose a class that is likely to have people with interests that are similar to yours. If you are successful, you will have proven to yourself that the belief *I cannot meet new people because I am in pain* is false. This experiment could improve your outlook and make you feel better.

Use the sheets *Thinking Patterns* and *Problematic Thought Patterns* at the end of this chapter to help you with your maladaptive thoughts. Feel free to make copies for your personal use. Filling out the sheets as you practice these techniques, especially in the beginning, is extremely important and will ensure that the benefits are all the more effective.

Summary

So what do you think? Are you willing to take a more active approach to managing your chronic pain? Try the techniques outlined in this chapter and see how effective they are for you. Start with one of the techniques (e.g., pacing) and apply it consistently. Once it has become a part of your regular routine, introduce another technique (e.g., diaphragmatic breathing or imagery), and so on. Alone, these individual techniques may not produce an overwhelming result, but as the number of added techniques starts to grow, you will most likely begin to see an improvement in your ability to manage your pain more effectively. The best part is that these techniques will help to put you in control of your pain, not the other way around!

A Word about Practice

As you know, practice is important when learning new skills. For example, when learning to play the piano or do ballroom dancing, beginners must practice in order to improve and excel. You simply can't learn to do some things overnight. The following exercises are designed to help you practice the techniques described in this chapter.

Distraction

1. Have you had experiences that allowed you to distract yourself from your pain? What were these experiences?

   _____

   _____

   _____

2. What are some things that you might try to take your mind off your pain?

   _____

   _____

   _____

3. During the day, when do you feel you could use distraction and give yourself a break from pain?

_____

_____

_____

Relaxation Questions

1. What words will you use as you breathe in and out?

"_____" when I inhale; "_____" when I exhale.

2. What images will be helpful for you in dealing with pain?

Place: _____

Sounds: _____

Sights: _____

Tastes: _____

Smells: _____

Relaxation Monitoring Sheet

Use this sheet to note the pain relief strategies you use (e.g., relaxation, belly breathing, distraction) and how helpful you find them.

0	1	2	3	4	5	6	7	8	9	10
very little help					moderately helpful				very helpful	

Day	Strategy	Minutes practiced	How helpful was the strategy?
Monday	Imagery	15	6
Tuesday	Belly breathing	5	8
	Watching a movie	120	10

Pacing

1. What activities do you tend to push yourself to do?

    _____

    _____

2. What activities do you feel could be broken up into smaller sections by taking scheduled rest periods?

    _____

    _____

3. How long do you think you should engage in these activities before resting?

    _____

    _____

4. How long do you think you should rest?

    _____

    _____

Thinking Patterns

Do you have any beliefs that may have a negative impact on the way you cope with pain? (See examples on pages 29–32). Write these down in the spaces below. Then rate the strength of each belief on a scale from 1 (mild belief) to 10 (strong belief).

Try substituting your problematic thought patterns with more realistic and adaptive thoughts. Many seniors, particularly those who feel very depressed, may need the assistance of a health care professional in overcoming maladaptive thoughts.

Problematic thought: "_____"

Rate the strength of this belief:

  1   2   3   4   5   6   7   8   9   10

Adaptive thought: "_____"

Rate the strength of this belief:

  1   2   3   4   5   6   7   8   9   10

Problematic thought: "_____"

Rate the strength of this belief:

  1   2   3   4   5   6   7   8   9   10

Adaptive thought: "_____"

Rate the strength of this belief:

  1   2   3   4   5   6   7   8   9   10

Problematic thought: "_____"

Rate the strength of this belief:

  1   2   3   4   5   6   7   8   9   10

Adaptive thought: "_____"

Rate the strength of this belief:

  1   2   3   4   5   6   7   8   9   10

Rating Sheet for Changing Problematic Thought Patterns

This sheet will help you to track the effectiveness of your efforts to change your problematic thought patterns. Use this sheet to monitor your mood before and after you substitute an adaptive thought.

Rate the intensity of your emotion(s) using the following scale:

1	2	3	4	5	6	7	8	9	10
	Weak				Moderate				Strong

Problematic thought	How you felt when you noticed the problematic thought	Rate the intensity of your feeling	Adaptive thought	Rate the intensity of your feeling after substituting the adaptive thought
I can't do anything if I have pain	*depressed*	8	*I am capable of doing things I enjoy despite having pain*	3

SANDRA M. LEFORT, RN, PHD
RONALD R. MARTIN, PHD, RD PSYCH.

CHAPTER FOUR

Pain and Emotion

Whenever your chronic pain flares up or worsens, do you begin to feel sad, helpless, or hopeless? If so, this is entirely understandable. Chronic pain can drain you of physical and emotional energy. In some cases, you may begin to feel down or depressed as you struggle with your ongoing pain. A depressed mood may, in turn, have a negative impact on your ability to manage your pain. This chapter will help you better understand the relationship between chronic pain and emotional states such as depression. More importantly, this chapter will provide you with a range of strategies that are designed to improve the way you feel.

This chapter also includes a discussion of the pain–depression cycle as well as ideas about how to deal with the blues. In addition, we discuss the signs of clinical depression and make recommendations about when to seek help with that disorder. At the end of the chapter you will find a number of useful exercises that have been found to be effective in improving a depressed mood.

The Pain-Depression Cycle

Everyone feels blue or gets down in the dumps at times. In fact, it is perfectly normal to feel sad or discouraged especially when you are dealing with a stressful problem such as chronic pain. Chronic pain and the stress that goes with it can lead to the blues or feelings of depression and fatigue. The more depressed and fatigued you are, the more pain you may feel. Greater pain leads to added stress, which may increase depression. And so the cycle continues.

39

Different Ways of Dealing with the Blues

There are a number of effective techniques, listed below, that are designed to break this cycle. These techniques help relieve feelings of depression and allow you to feel good about yourself. You may find that when you are feeling good, you are already making regular use of several of these techniques. However, the challenge is to begin using these techniques when you first start to feel depressed. This is difficult because when you feel down in the dumps you may want to give up or you may not have the energy to try to make things better. This is the time you need these techniques most!

Having a variety of mood-enhancing techniques is important for older adults, because not all seniors are the same. People age differently and have different preferences. Some people will find certain techniques more useful than others.

As you explore different methods, remember that it is helpful to take small steps. Try just one or two methods at a time and give them the opportunity to have an effect. You will have a better chance to succeed, because smaller changes can be more easily incorporated into your everyday life. If you try to introduce too many changes all at once, you may feel overwhelmed and you will be more likely to experience setbacks.

Examine your thoughts about yourself and the world around you. The way you think about yourself and the world around you is related to your mood. People who are depressed tend to think of themselves and their worlds in negative, pessimistic ways. They sometimes convince themselves that they are not worthwhile people. Seniors with depression sometimes say things to themselves similar to the following:

> *"I didn't accomplish anything in my life. I'm a failure."*
> *"Now that I'm a widow(er), I can never be happy."*
> *"My whole body is aching; I can't accomplish anything any more."*

These kinds of thoughts are associated with depression, which contributes to chronic pain (e.g., by causing social isolation and by increasing the focus on pain). When you have negative thoughts like these and believe them to be true, it naturally follows that you will experience debilitating emotions. It is important to realize that views about oneself, such as the ones above, tend to be incorrect no matter how firmly a person holds them. Things are rarely so black and white.

Let's take the example of the belief *"Now that I'm a widow(er), I can never be happy."* If you enjoyed a good relationship with a spouse who has passed away, it may be true that you have lost a great deal. Remember that the loss of a loved one is part of life. In order to cope successfully with loss, we must remember that there are always many worthwhile and enjoyable things in life. Friends and family members contribute to the enjoyment of our lives as do hobbies, travel, and many other activities. Focusing on what you have and your options to improve the quality of your life will help you adjust to setbacks far more effectively than thinking, *"I can never be happy now."* Instead of choosing to be fatalistic, try telling yourself something like the following:

> *"Although the loss of my loved one is truly very sad and I will never forget him/her, I must go on with life and find those things that will make my life more enjoyable and worthwhile. Perhaps I will pick up a hobby I abandoned but once enjoyed. I could also try to get in touch with old friends I have not seen for a long time. I will try to think of other things that will improve the quality of my life."*

Take some time to look at the things you say to yourself in your private thoughts. If you notice that you often think negatively about yourself and the world around you, it may be helpful to target such thoughts and substitute them with more realistic, adaptive statements. This change in your thought patterns may ultimately help you feel better emotionally and physically. At the end of the chapter, you will find an exercise (pages 48–49) to assist you in identifying maladaptive thoughts. This general approach has been developed by famous psychotherapists such as Dr. Aaron Beck. The exercise builds upon the work that was discussed in Chapter 3. Be sure to read Chapter 3 and complete the exercises there before working on the sheets at the end of this chapter.

Acknowledge and examine your negative emotions. Sometimes, trying to sort out your feelings and pinpoint the source of your depression can be helpful. Depression might be a cover for other emotions such as anxiety, anger, guilt, or frustration—emotions that you may feel uncomfortable with. Once you acknowledge your feelings, you can begin to figure out what to do about them. When we don't acknowledge our emotions, finding a solution can be difficult.

Allow yourself to experience your emotions. Face it: You feel crummy. Don't belittle yourself for feeling blue. It is part of the pain–depression cycle. Learning to adjust to, and cope with, a problem like chronic pain is understandably difficult.

Simplify a complex task. Sometimes you may find yourself feeling overwhelmed by even the most uncomplicated task. This may lower your confidence and leave you feeling helpless. Try breaking down larger, more complex projects into smaller, more manageable tasks. Remember the old saying: *"A journey of a thousand miles begins with a single step!"*

A man who participated in one of our pain management groups had a room in his house that had been messy for years. He considered the task of cleaning the room to be overwhelming and kept putting off doing anything about it. We suggested to him that he dedicate 15 minutes a day to the task and no more. By breaking down the task into *baby steps* he was able to clean the room completely in a month. The project became manageable because he focused on one small step at a time. At the end, he felt better about himself and even decided to redecorate the room, which became a favorite place for him to read, listen to music, relax, and watch television. We advised him to spend about 5 to 10 minutes a day ensuring that the room was neat, and this worked very well for him.

Pick up a pen or a box of crayons. A great way to express your feelings is to write them down or even draw pictures of them. Sit down with a pen and write or use colored crayons to sketch whatever comes to mind using the colors that best express how you feel. You might be surprised at the insight you gain into your emotions.

Do not assume that others have bad intentions. Sometimes we feel depressed because we have misunderstood someone's words or actions. Before jumping to conclusions, consider that there are many ways to interpret the actions of others. For example, we may assume that someone does not spend much time with us because he or she does not enjoy our company. In fact, this individual may be preoccupied, anxious about a personal matter, or simply rushed.

Talk it out and then do things with others. It is always helpful to share your feelings with someone else you care about and trust. But don't leave it at that. Do things with friends and family—eat out, go to the movies, go shopping, or take a walk.

Keep being active. Hanging around the house could add to your depression. Pace your activities so that you can be as active as possible—take a walk, visit a friend, play a game of cards, become a volunteer. Variety is important. Turning on the television is not being active!

Exercise. Research tells us that regular exercise may be the single most effective thing you can do to overcome the blues and fatigue. Most people benefit from exercise when using a program that is appropriate for their physical condition. The topic of exercise is addressed in detail in Chapter 6.

Take pride in your appearance. Get dressed in your favorite clothes. Women, put on makeup if you normally wear it. Men, shave and get a new haircut. Looking good may help you feel good.

Search your memory for fun things to do. The best way to pick an activity is to start by jotting down a list of things you used to enjoy doing. Your sense of enjoment may return if you make an effort to rediscover these things. Give yourself a chance. Pick one of your old activities— or even choose a new one—and give it a try. Remember, however, that when people have the blues or are depressed, they do not instantly begin to enjoy the things that they once loved doing. But most people find that if they persist in introducing additional, possibly pleasant activities to their schedules, their enjoyment increases within a few weeks and their mood improves. Remember also that sometimes people with the blues tend to underestimate the enjoyment that an activity is likely to give them. Many of our clients are surprised to find that any scheduled activities turn out to be more enjoyable than they anticipated. At the end of this chapter (pages 50–53) you will find exercises and monitoring sheets designed to help you increase the pleasant activities in your life. Together with his collaborators, Dr. Lewinsohn, a well-known depression researcher, has used such exercises and monitoring sheets to show that people can often overcome major depression by systematically increasing the number of enjoyable pursuits in their lives.

Feel free to copy and use the **Weekly Mood/Activity Monitoring Sheet.** This sheet not only allows you to *predict* how much enjoyment you expect from each planned activity; it *lets you rate how pleasant the activity actually was.* You may be surprised to discover that such planned events bring you more pleasure than you could have predicted. You may also find that this is especially true if you persist with these pleasurable activities. Increasing the enjoyable pursuits in your life should go a long way toward helping you improve your mood.

Have a good laugh. There is nothing like a good laugh to make any situation seem lighter. In his book *Anatomy of An Illness*, Norman Cousins wrote about the great benefits of humor and laughter in healing our bodies and minds. For starters, why not rent a funny movie one afternoon when you are feeling blue? Better yet, get someone to watch it with you. Laughter is contagious!

Slow down. Life can be hectic even with chronic pain. Are you over-scheduling activities, exhausting yourself, and then collapsing? Maybe you need more time. If so, you may need to reorganize your priorities and think about more realistic goals.

Avoid making major life decisions. Don't make momentous changes in your life when you are down in the dumps. Wait until you are feeling better. You don't want to make the wrong decision. That would only drag you down further.

Join a group. Get involved in structured activities. Join a group at your church, synagogue, or mosque, join a discussion group or a hobby club, or take a course.

Get a pet or a plant. Recent research indicates that pets can help us cope better with stress in our lives. Even plants can affect us positively. Things that need care and draw attention away from thinking too much about ourselves can make us feel better. Remember that, in general, smaller pets are easier to manage than larger ones. Walking a big dog on an icy street in the winter could increase your chances of a fall.

Watch your alcohol intake. Are you drinking alcohol to forget your troubles or to decrease your pain? Alcohol is a downer. For most people, one drink a day is not a problem. But if your body and mind are not free of alcohol most of the time, you are having trouble with this drug. Seek help.

44

Watch what you eat. Nutrition has a definite effect on emotions. What we eat is connected with how we feel about ourselves. When we are depressed, we tend to pass over foods we know are good for us and instead choose high-fat junkfood or candies. Good nutrition is especially important when dealing with the stress of chronic pain. Unless your doctor tells you otherwise, you may find it helpful to cut down on stimulants such as caffeine *(see Chapter 8)*.

Check your medications. Some medications taken for chronic pain and other health problems can themselves make depression worse. These include tranquilizers, some analgesics (painkillers), certain sleeping pills, and other drugs. Check with your pharmacist or call your doctor to find out if depression is a side effect of your medications. If you really need medications, your doctor may be able to prescribe other similar drugs that will not affect your mood. Remember, don't discontinue a prescription drug without first talking to your doctor. There may be important reasons why you are on the drug, or there may be with-drawal reactions. So, always call your doctor first.

Use the forms at the end of this chapter to help you plan more pleasant activities and to start replacing any counter-productive thoughts with more adaptive ones. Feel free to make copies of the exercises and other materials there for your personal use.

Signs of Depression: Knowing When to Get Help

As we mentioned earlier, everyone occasionally feels unhappy, and it is normal to have periods when you are blue, especially when you have a problem such as chronic pain. For most of us, these feelings pass in a few hours or days or may even last a week or two. Eventually, though, most of us see that things are not all black—rays of sunshine glimmer through the clouds of our depressed feelings and we begin to feel better.

However, for some people with chronic pain, feelings of depression do not go away. These people do not see any rays of hope and carry a double burden: they are trying to cope with chronic pain and are also struggling with unrelenting depression.

One of the difficulties of having chronic pain is recognizing when you are suffering from depression. This is not always easy because some of the signs of depression are also signs of chronic pain. These include sleep disturbance, irritability, and trouble concentrating. Scientists think that an imbalance of certain chemicals in the brain (such as serotonin) may be involved in both depression and chronic pain. This explains why some of the signs of depression are also signs of chronic pain. But this does *not* mean that if you have chronic pain you must be chronically depressed.

Many people tend to think that depression is part and parcel of chronic pain. They say things like, "He has a right to be depressed! Look at all he's going through." However, it is important to keep in mind that chronic pain does not necessarily lead to depression. In fact, we are regularly confronted with examples of individuals who are faced with ongoing, major challenges yet still manage to adapt and carry on (for example, Christopher Reeve, after the accident that left him paralyzed and dependent on mechanical breathing, had a meaningful and joyful life).

The following are some signs of depression. You probably have experienced several of them if you suffer from chronic pain or take pain medications.

- Feelings of depression most of the time nearly every day.
- Decreased interest or pleasure in all or most of your everyday activities.
- Substantial weight loss or weight gain, or a significant increase or decrease in your appetite nearly every day.
- Sleeping much more or much less than usual or consistently waking up earlier than usual in the morning. Sleep disturbances, especially trouble getting to sleep and frequent waking, are common in those with chronic pain.
- Excessive activity or greatly reduced activity levels nearly every day. These changes are significant enough that other people would probably notice them.
- Fatigue or lack of energy nearly every day.
- Feelings of worthlessness or excessive or unrealistic guilt.
- Lowered ability to think or concentrate nearly every day. Remember that concentration may be affected by pain and by pain medication.

◎ Thinking that life is not worth living. If you have had recurring thoughts of death or suicide, get help from your doctor or psychologist. *Do not delay. Call for help immediately.* These feelings do not mean you are crazy. Chronic pain is a difficult problem, but you can learn to cope with it. Your depression can be treated. Talking with an understanding person and getting the help you need will see you through this period.

Are some of these signs familiar to you? If you experience a few of these feelings and they are mild, you can do many things to help change them. Try some of the suggestions we have already discussed.

You do not need to have all of the above symptoms to be clinically depressed. But if you have had four or more of these signs continuously for weeks and nothing helps, you may be clinically depressed. You may not feel like making the effort to get help, but it is important that you do so. Tell one person you trust and confide in your doctor. They can help you get the help you need.

Summary

Pain can increase *the blues* or feelings of depression, and depression can increase pain. If you experience chronic pain and feel depressed, remember that there are many things you can do to improve your wellbeing. Having chronic pain does not mean that you must also suffer unrelenting depression.

A good place to start is by asking yourself if there are any activities or hobbies that you used to enjoy in the past but have since given up. If it is possible for you to take part in these activities (perhaps with some minor modifications), consider reintroducing them into your everyday life. If it is no longer possible for you to do these things, then consider the other strategies outlined in this chapter. In fact, you should try more than one of these approaches at a time to see which ones work best for you. Finally, if you have signs of clinical depression that are not getting better, seek help from your doctor, psychologist, nurse practitioner, or other qualified health care professional as soon as possible.

Examining Your Thoughts

Step 1: Take some time to reflect on the thoughts you have about yourself and the world around you. Do you commonly say/ think maladaptive things? Here are some examples of the kind of negative thoughts you should avoid:

- ⊚ *"The world is a horrible place for a senior citizen."*
- ⊚ *"Now that I'm older, I can't do anything."*
- ⊚ *"Nobody would ever want to spend time with me."*
- ⊚ *"It's impossible for me to learn how to do anything new. "*

Step 2: Take a moment to record your maladaptive thoughts and beliefs below. If this is difficult, pay attention to the thoughts going through your mind when you are feeling low.

_____

_____

_____

Step 3: *Dispute* your maladaptive thoughts and beliefs and substitute them with adaptive, positive ones.

Although you may firmly believe the negative thoughts and beliefs you recorded, they are likely to be incorrect. Most things are not black or white. It is important to dispute your maladaptive thoughts and beliefs by looking at things objectively and rationally. This process is demonstrated in the following example: Maladaptive thought: *"I am a total failure."*

Dispute the thought: *"Although everyone experiences some failures in life, no one is a total failure. Every human being accomplishes certain things in his or her life. These vary from person to person but include things such as raising children or helping people by fulfilling one's primary role. A carpenter builds houses where people live, a teacher instructs students how to read* *and write, an airline pilot transports thousands to their loved ones, a gardener plants trees and beautiful flowers. Virtually everyone has helped other people in some fashion throughout their lives. No one is ever a total failure or a total success."*

Substitute an adaptive thought: *"I have accomplished many worthwhile things."* (List the things you have accomplished.)

Step 4: In the future, monitor your thoughts and speech for existing maladaptive thoughts and beliefs and for new ones that may arise. Whenever you recognize a maladaptive thought or belief, dispute it and then substitute a more adaptive one.

Using the following table, list your maladaptive thoughts on the left and then dispute each one in the space to the right. Feel free to make copies of the table for your personal use.

Maladaptive Thought/Belief	Dispute the Thought/Belief	Substitute an Adaptive Thought/Belief
Example: "I am a total failure."	"No one is a total failure. Everyone accomplishes things in life. My accomplishments include providing a home for my children."	"I have accomplished many worthwhile things and have struggled with other things. This is what life is all about."

Potentially Enjoyable Activities

Search your memory for fun things to do. Researchers have discovered that people who feel sad or depressed can improve their mood and feel better simply by increasing the numbers of pleasant activities in which they engage. If you feel depressed or down, you may find it difficult to initiate such activities. Patients sometimes tell us things like, *"Why should I go to a movie? I know I won't enjoy it. I used to like going to movies but I don't any more."* While it may be true that activities that used to be enjoyable no longer seem fun, getting into a routine of doing more things that used to be pleasurable can increase your quality of life. It may be hard to take the first step, but once you do, there is typically a payoff in terms of improved mood.

Researchers have also found that people who feel unhappy often tend to underestimate the amount of pleasure that various activities are likely to give them. You may feel skeptical about this, but we are not asking you to take our word for it. Instead, we want you to treat this like an experiment. Try it for a week or even a day and see if this approach results in a greater amount of enjoyment and a better quality of life.

Step 1: Select a variety of activities that you used to enjoy but no longer find pleasurable and list them below. These things can take just a brief amount of time (e.g., playing music, calling a friend on the phone), or they can be more time-intensive (e.g., getting your hair cut, going to a movie, playing cards).

_____

_____

_____

_____

Step 2: Continue to build on the list of potentially pleasurable activities by looking over the list below. Mark the items that could potentially give you a sense of pleasure:

___ Spending time with family.

___ Taking grandchildren to places or participating with them in activities they enjoy (e.g., a trip to the circus, the park, or a museum or science center).

___ Going to the movies.

___ Getting a massage.

___ Visiting a spa.

___ Taking a walk.

___ Swimming or enjoying a soak in a hot tub.

___ Stretching.

___ Sitting in the yard.

___ Enjoying the sunset.

___ Calling or writing to a friend.

___ Going out for coffee.

___ Eating at a restaurant.

___ Visiting a second-hand store.

___ Going to a football game.

___ Spending an hour at the public library.

___ Visiting an art gallery.

___ Taking in a live show (e.g., the theater, the symphony).

___ Joining a club.

___ Volunteering at a hospital or museum.

___ Signing up for an interesting class (e.g., woodworking, drawing, T'ai Chi, yoga, computers).

___ Going fishing.

___ Planning a trip to the lake.

___ Buying or borrowing a book or a CD.

___ Shopping for new clothes.

___ Gardening.

___ Sewing or knitting.

___ Cleaning up around the house (e.g., tidying a closet).

___ Looking at photograph albums.

___ Listening to music.

___ Cooking dinner or baking a cake.

___ Playing cards.

___ Challenging your spouse or friend to a board game.

Step 3: Select four or five activities to do over the next week (activities that you were *not* going to do otherwise).

Step 4: Use the form on the following page. Mark the pleasant activities that you engaged in each day. Before each activity write down the amount of pleasure that you expect to have. After each one (at the end of the day before retiring), make a note of how much pleasure you actually experienced. Over several weeks, most people find that the pleasant activities become increasingly enjoyable and that their mood experienced through the day is related to the amount and quality of pleasant activities that they engage in.

Weekly Mood/Activity Monitoring Sheets

Rate how much pleasure you *expected* or *actually had* from each activity using this scale:

| 1 | 2 | 3 | 4 | 5 | 6 | 7 | 8 | 9 | 10 |

no pleasure   *maximum pleasure*

Day of Week	Activity	How much pleasure you expected from this activity	How much pleasure you actually had from this activity
Monday	Talking to a friend	4	7
Monday	Going to a movie	5	8

CHAPTER FIVE

Social Support, Loneliness, and Pain

Larry

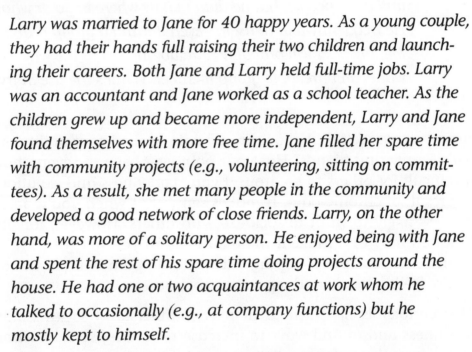

Larry was married to Jane for 40 happy years. As a young couple, they had their hands full raising their two children and launching their careers. Both Jane and Larry held full-time jobs. Larry was an accountant and Jane worked as a school teacher. As the children grew up and became more independent, Larry and Jane found themselves with more free time. Jane filled her spare time with community projects (e.g., volunteering, sitting on committees). As a result, she met many people in the community and developed a good network of close friends. Larry, on the other hand, was more of a solitary person. He enjoyed being with Jane and spent the rest of his spare time doing projects around the house. He had one or two acquaintances at work whom he talked to occasionally (e.g., at company functions) but he mostly kept to himself.

When the children left home to go off to college, Larry took on more responsibilities at work to keep busy. The years flew by and Larry and Jane decided to retire. Shortly after retirement, Larry developed a degenerative condition that affected his knees. At times, the pain was unbearable. Surgery helped the problem and allowed him to continue walking, but he was left to cope with the chronic pain.

Undaunted, Larry and Jane decided to make the most of their retirement. They planned to travel together and spend their time in various leisurely recreational pursuits. Tragically, Jane passed away before these plans could be realized. Larry found himself on his own. The first few years following Jane's death were very hard for Larry. However, he moved through the grieving process and learned a lot about himself along the way. One of the things he realized was that he was lonely. He socialized with a few people (his old acquaintances from work) but felt that these relationships were largely unsatisfying. His children told him to get out there and meet people, but he didn't know where to go or what to do. He frequently told himself, "Even if I find a group that interests me, my pain will probably flare up and get in the way. No one wants an unreliable group member. What's the use in trying?"

Have you ever felt that your chronic pain limited your ability to socialize with family and friends? Has your pain ever been so severe that it made it difficult for others to be around you? Loneliness and isolation may be the result of chronic pain. It makes sense that when you're in pain, you are less likely to want to socialize with others. However, loneliness and isolation may also make it more difficult for you to deal with the consequences of your pain. Coping with chronic pain is more difficult when you're feeling lonely and separated from others.

This chapter is intended to help you understand social isolation and loneliness and to find ways to increase rewarding social exchanges. We will discuss the difference between social isolation and social loneliness. We will also examine the consequences that loneliness can have for health and well-being and review strategies for reducing its effects.

Take some time to think about the social network you have developed over the course of your adult life. Think of the times you've spent with your family, friends and other acquaintances. Have you noticed changes? As an older adult, what changes have you noticed regarding the size of your social network, the people you spend time with, and the nature of those relationships?

Social Isolation versus Loneliness

In many cases, as people age, the size of social networks tends to decrease due to naturally occurring events such as retirement, illness, the deaths of loved ones, and limitations in hearing, vision, and mobility. Have you found this to be the case in your life? In a discussion of the changing social environments of seniors, it is important to define two similar, yet distinct concepts. The first is *social isolation*. Social isolation refers to the *number* of personal contacts you have. If you have few relationships with others (e.g., relatives, friends, neighbors, co-workers), you may be socially isolated. In contrast, the second concept, *social loneliness*, describes a *feeling of dissatisfaction* with the quantity and/or quality of your social relationships. Social loneliness often occurs following the death of a long-time spouse, partner, or friend.

People sometimes don't feel the need to be around others and simply *choose* to be alone. These people may be *socially isolated* according to the technical definition, but they aren't lonely. On the other hand, people who are dissatisfied with their lack of social contacts are experiencing *social loneliness*. A person can have many social contacts and still feel lonely if the relationships are not satisfying or rewarding.

Remember Larry from the vignette at the start of the chapter? Did he experience social isolation, social loneliness, or both?

Overall, Larry experienced both social isolation (he had very few personal relationships with others) and social loneliness (he felt that his connections with others were unsatisfying).

Take a moment to think about what it would be like to experience social isolation and/or loneliness. What other things might go hand-in-hand with these problems? Researchers have found that social isolation and/or social loneliness have been associated with *anxiety and depression, suicide* (in extreme cases involving severe depression), and *greater use of health care services.* The presence of social isolation and loneliness is also associated with *lower ratings in both overall health and life satisfaction, and a greater number of chronic conditions* including mobility and sensory problems (e.g., people with hearing difficulties may have greater difficulty participating in social conversations), low back or abdominal pain, headache, peptic ulcers, respiratory disorders, diabetes, coronary heart disease, and arteriosclerosis.

Clearly, chronic pain problems can increase the probability of social isolation and loneliness since people may find it physically difficult to go to places where socialization is more likely (e.g., visiting a friend's home, joining and attending a social club or meeting for a game of cards). On the other hand, social activity and social support can distract people from pain problems and help them improve their quality of life. Carefully pacing oneself through an increasing number of social activities can make it easier for an older adult with pain to expand his or her social network. The technique of pacing, discussed in more detail in Chapter 3, is used to balance activity and rest through a consistent and realistic schedule. Many older adults with pain conditions find they can become more active, without having more pain, by using the pacing technique.

One important research finding is that, for older adults, loneliness seems to be associated with the *quality* of social relationships rather than the *quantity*. Therefore, the average older adult might feel less lonely by cultivating a smaller number of more emotionally satisfying relationships rather than a larger number of less meaningful ones. However, in general, meeting new people will increase the probability of developing truly meaningful relationships.

In addition to this general finding, gender differences have been shown to play a role in social isolation and loneliness. Some studies affirm that women are more likely to express social loneliness than men. This may not be surprising given that women tend to live longer than men and therefore are more likely to be widowed and to live alone. In addition, women usually have larger social support systems than men which help them deal with emotional difficulties such as loneliness. Men typically have smaller social networks. Following the death of a partner, men may be more prone to social loneliness.

How did Larry and Jane differ in their social patterns throughout their marriage? As you may recall from the vignette at the start of the chapter, Jane filled her free time with activities that allowed her to interact with others and build relationships. In contrast, Larry preferred more solitary activities, and he tended to socialize infrequently (usually with co-workers). After Jane passed away, his limited social connections left him feeling isolated and lonely.

As mentioned earlier, social isolation and social loneliness are linked to various chronic health problems. Sometimes health problems (e.g., chronic pain) can lead to social isolation and loneliness, and some researchers have proposed that loneliness can have a negative effect on health problems. In addition to these two possibilities, other factors such as depression may influence both social isolation/loneliness and health problems.

> **IMPORTANT:** *If you are extremely isolated and lonely and get little satisfaction from the quality or quantity of your social contacts, try the techniques below. If you remain isolated and lonely, seek help from your doctor or psychologist. Over time, severe isolation and social loneliness may lead to feelings of depression. Talk with your doctor about how to address this problem.*

Find and Foster Relationships

To reduce social isolation, you must first increase the number of your social contacts. There are many sources for extra social contact including family, friends, neighbors, former colleagues and co-workers, and volunteer organizations.

However, if social loneliness is a problem, it is necessary to seek out and foster relationships with others whom you find satisfying and rewarding. Try calling your local seniors' center for information about various groups and programs (e.g., exercise or walking groups, discussion clubs, or continuing education classes for seniors). If you make an effort to connect, you will likely find others in the same situation! Many seniors find that pets provide good companionship. The Internet is also a means for seniors with computers to communicate with others (e.g., via email). This would be especially relevant for those seniors who are frail and homebound or for older adults who are otherwise isolated or living in rural areas.

If you experience social isolation or loneliness and you would like to mingle more with others, try going to places that will increase your chances of interacting with others who may share similar interests. Seniors' centers and fitness or leisure organizations are excellent places to meet other people. Frequently, courses (e.g., cooking, pottery, carpentry) are offered to seniors at these facilities, along with social gatherings and fitness groups (e.g., bridge clubs, walking or sightseeing groups). Most cities and many smaller towns will have facilities such as leisure centers that offer these kinds of services to seniors. Another option may be to join support groups related to the health problem you experience (e.g., arthritis, diabetes). Several organizations listed starting on page 186 of this book either offer such support groups or will be able to provide you with relevant information.

Making Small Talk

It may have been a while since you met new people, and it can be intimidating. Below, we list some ideas about how to make small talk.

1. Read up on things you enjoy and want to discuss with others. Topics can include cookbooks, newspaper or magazine articles. If you intend to join a group, read about your chosen topic beforehand. If you don't enjoy reading, watch a television program or listen to the radio.

2. Practice retelling a story you have read or heard on television or on the radio. You can even do this by yourself. If you are especially anxious, consider joining a local Toastmasters group (visit their web site at *http://www.toastmasters.org/*). People who want to improve their communication skills (e.g., because they feel anxious) often join Toastmasters where they practice speaking in a supportive group environment. Most people we know who have joined Toastmasters say that the experience is most enjoyable.

3. Keep a journal of interesting things that happen to you or that you see on a daily basis and review these before you go out.

4. Make a list of any topics that come to mind and think about what you might have to say about them. Subjects might include the weather, sports, animals, department stores, or news events.

5. Try something new and share this experience with new people you meet.

6. Practice chatting with people you come across in your daily life, including your neighbors. When chatting with others, be sure you take time to listen and ask questions. Make a list of questions you feel comfortable asking someone new. *"How long have you been coming here?"* or *"What do you like about this place?"* or *"What other things do you like to do?"*

7. Once you get to know people, host your own gathering. This can be something as simple as having people over or meeting somewhere for tea.

Challenge Negative Thoughts

If you are not used to maintaining a satisfying social life, the task of overcoming problems with social isolation or loneliness might seem very challenging. Some older adults may even feel that making new contacts is too difficult or even impossible, especially given their problems with chronic pain. The following are examples of the negative things some people say to themselves, each of them followed by a possible rebuttal:

Negative thought: *"My pain prevents me from socializing."*

Rebuttal: *"Pain can make socialization a bit more difficult but, if I pace myself, I can do more. I can also talk to friends and family over the phone. Connecting with other people will take my mind off the pain and could help me feel better."*

Negative thought: *"I would be embarrassed if others knew about my chronic pain."*

Rebuttal: *"Many people have problems with pain. Most everyone understands that, and there is nothing embarrassing about it."*

Negative thought: *"The people I might meet probably wouldn't understand my limitations."*

Rebuttal: *"There may be people who will not understand my limitations. However, many others will, and I can choose the company of those who are most understanding."*

Negative thought: *"If I join a group and I can't attend a meeting, I would feel as if I'd be letting everyone down. Why start something you can't commit to 100%?"*

Rebuttal: *"Many people join groups and take classes with varying degrees of commitment. Some are less committed than others. When taking a recreational class or picking up a new hobby, I can do whatever I feel comfortable doing."*

Sometimes, believing a rebuttal might require a *behavioral experiment* (i.e., trying to find out for yourself if the statement is true). Chapter 3 gives more information on how to set up *a behavioral experiment* designed to help you change such beliefs. There is nothing more convincing than finding out for yourself!

After Jane died, Larry was socially isolated (i.e., he had very few social contacts) and he was lonely (i.e., he was unhappy with the quantity and quality of his interpersonal relationships). So he decided he would do something about it by getting involved in his community. At first he was hesitant because he thought that his pain would prevent him from being a reliable member of any group. But much to his surprise, he found organizations that were flexible about attendance. He also adjusted his attitude by telling himself, "I will do everything I can to manage my pain, but occasionally I won't be able to attend a meeting. That doesn't mean that I should scrap the idea of joining a group. I'd be cheating myself out of getting to know other interesting people."

Larry joined two community organizations that interested him. He dreaded those first few outings. But he kept telling himself, "Just try it" and "You have nothing to lose." After getting over the initial jitters, he found himself looking forward to getting out. In both organizations, he volunteered to fill the role of treasurer, putting his strong accounting skills to use, which gave him a sense of self-worth.

Over time, he realized he was spending more time with numbers than he was with people! So, he changed his strategy. He passed on his role as treasurer to another person and eventually became an events coordinator. Soon, he was meeting a variety of interesting people. Among these new social contacts, Larry discovered a few special people whom he loved to socialize with. Larry still enjoyed his time alone, but whenever he wanted to be with friends, he always had people to call. He knew that Jane would be proud of his efforts to carry on and connect with others.

Summary

As you read through this chapter, did you recognize in yourself any of the signs of loneliness or isolation? If you did and you feel unhappy because of it, we encourage you to take action to improve your levels of social support. Pain problems can sometimes contribute to loneliness and social isolation.

As you begin to try to increase your social circle, remember to be patient. Sometimes it takes time for social relationships to form. Just as a gardener must plant many seeds and cultivate them, you must allow developing social relationships to blossom naturally. The end result is well worth it!

Social Isolation and Loneliness Problem-Solving Sheet

1. Would you like to have more contact with:

    ○ Family   ○ Friends   ○ Neighbors

    ○ Former coworkers   ○ Volunteer organizations   ○ Social support groups

2. Strategies you can use to increase your contact:

    ○ Phone   ○ Write

    ○ Arrange to have coffee or a meal outside of your home

    ○ Arrange an activity inside the home

    ○ Invite someone into your home for coffee

    ○ Arrange an activity outside the home

    List your own strategies below:

    _____

    _____

    _____

3. Would you like to join a new group? What types of groups interest you?

    ○ Walking   ○ Swimming   ○ Exercise

    ○ Health   ○ Cards   ○ Crafts

    ○ Cooking/baking   ○ Animals   ○ Painting

    ○ Computer   ○ Bridge   ○ Pottery

    ○ Carpentry   ○ Travel   ○ Gardening

    ○ Other _____

4. Look up the contact information for your local leisure center, museum, college/university, senior center, or health care organization and ask for information.

5. What thoughts do you have that prevent you from getting involved?

    ○ *"My pain prevents me from socializing."*

    ○ *"I would be embarrassed if others knew about my chronic pain."*

    ○ *"Other people I might meet probably wouldn't understand my limitations."*

    ○ *"If I join a group and I can't attend a meeting, I would feel as if I would be letting everyone down. Why start something you can't commit to 100%?"*

    "I am too old to start meeting new friends now."

    Other thoughts: _____

6. Write down your rebuttal to these negative thoughts *(see the examples earlier in this chapter)*.

7. If you can't think of a rebuttal, try out a behavioral experiment to see if your thoughts are in fact true (refer to Chapter 3 for more information on behavioral experiments).

    ○ Tell someone about your chronic pain. Is it really as embarrassing as you imagine? Does this person also experience pain?

    ○ Tell someone about your limitations (e.g., the need to stand frequently) and ask for suggestions on how you might improve the situation. Does this person really feel this is a problem, or can he or she help you overcome it?

NANCY K. TURNER, MSC
ELIZABETH L. HARRISON, PHD, BPT
ROBERT MCCULLOCH, PHD
RONALD R. MARTIN, PHD, RD PSYCH.

CHAPTER SIX

The Role of Exercise in Seniors' Lives

The exercises and activities in this section are suggestions only and may not be appropriate for your specific needs. Exercises and activities should be modified or deleted as necessary to fit your individual needs. Talk to your health professional before starting a new physical activity or exercise program. In some cases your physician may recommend that you come in for a more thorough medical examination, or he or she may suggest you see a physical therapist to help you select the right exercises based on your condition and function *(please also see the disclaimer in the front pages of this book).*

Have you ever thought or been told that you shouldn't exercise if you have chronic pain? In most cases, regular exercise is beneficial for seniors with ongoing pain problems. This might seem counterintuitive. You might think, *"I can't exercise. I have a chronic pain problem. Exercising will just make it worse."* This chapter will show you that supervised exercise that is approved by a qualified health professional, such as a physician or physiotherapist, may help you manage your pain more effectively. It could also help to reduce the risk of falling and injuring yourself.

In addition to outlining the importance and benefits of regular exercise, this chapter will provide you with essential information about the basic components of a well-rounded exercise program. Specifically, this chapter will review the benefits of physical activity, the importance of exercise in pain management, and the elements of general fitness. It will set out a program of physical activity including warm-up activities, aerobic exercises, strengthening and stretching exercises, and cool-down activities.

Toward the end of this chapter (pages 101–102) you will see brief descriptions of other forms of exercise (such as T'ai Chi and yoga) that many older adults have found beneficial.

Benefits of Activity

There are numerous benefits to maintaining an active lifestyle that includes physical exercise. Consider this quote from R.J. Shephard's *Aging, Physical Activity and Health*:

> *There is no known pharmacological remedy that can safely and*
> *effectively reduce a person's biological age and enhance his or*
> *her quality-adjusted life expectancy. Regular physical activity*
> *has the potential to do this and more.*

Consistent with what the first Director of the National Institute on Aging once said, if all of the benefits of regular physical activity could be put into a pill, it would be the most powerful medication known. Keeping in mind the unique individual health and fitness characteristics that each of us possesses, regular physical activity has the potential to be of great benefit to all older adults. Well-known benefits include lower blood pressure, weight control, maintenance of bone density, improved joint mobility, and increased strength. Regular activity is also valuable for stress management, improving energy levels, and improving one's ability to relax. It also provides opportunities for socialization.

Regular physical exercise has a positive influence on nearly all the body's systems: cardiovascular, respiratory, musculoskeletal, and endocrine. Exercise reduces the risk of cancer, stroke, osteoporosis, and diabetes.

Higher levels of physical activity are associated with better cognitive functioning. In fact, researchers now propose that regular exercise may help to enhance mental performance and even protect the brain from certain types of decline. At a minimum, regular physical activity can be helpful in maintaining self-esteem, independence, and an overall feeling of well-being. It is never too late to start a program of exercise and physical activity!

Exercise and Chronic Pain

Exercise is essential in the management of chronic pain. This may seem the opposite of what you would expect. You might expect that limiting your physical activity and not exercising would allow you to avoid pain and discomfort. While this seems to make sense, the fact is that reduced physical activity over long periods of time will lead to joint stiffness and weaker muscles. This in turn will cause further pain and physical decline. A prolonged sedentary lifestyle may also be associated with an increased risk of falls. Thus, getting regular exercise will allow you to manage your pain more effectively and reduce your risk of injury.

If you are thinking about starting or modifying an exercise program, remember that any regimen of physical activity should be designed to meet your needs, skills, interests, and capabilities. The general goal for physical activity programs designed for older adults is to help boost energy levels and add enjoyment and enthusiasm to everyday life. Even the most simple, basic movement patterns or the most elementary exercises can be the start of a helpful, positive daily program of physical activity.

Getting Ready: When, Where, What to Wear, and Other Considerations

Timing. When starting an exercise program, think about the best time of day to exercise. If you have more stiffness in the morning it is helpful to do some easy exercises to help you get moving (this by itself often reduces pain). Moreover, if you get tired at certain times of the day it is helpful to consider the relative timing of your exercise program. In some cases a bit of easy exercise when you are tired may help you feel refreshed. This having been said, more prolonged or intense exercises should not be done when you are fatigued because it is more difficult to be motivated and to do your exercises safely and appropriately. Be sure to discuss the timing of the exercise with your physical therapist or other health professional.

Clothing. If you have not been exercising regularly in the past, you may not have clothes that are suitable for exercise. Be sure to wear comfortable clothes as well as footwear that is specifically made for exercise and provides good support.

Location. It is important that you feel good when you exercise. Select a location with a comfortable temperature and good ventilation (i.e., not too cold or too hot). Make sure the tread on your shoes will prevent slipping. Exercise on firm but not soft surfaces. If you have problems with balance, make sure you exercise in an area where there is something to hold on to when you are standing in case you lose your balance.

Consult a physical therapist. This chapter has been developed for older adults who live independently in their own homes and have chronic pain that is primarily musculoskeletal in nature (e.g., back problems, arthritis). You should make sure that your exercise program is designed to accommodate any functional limitations you may have (e.g., pain, limited joint mobility, or decreased balance). A physical therapist can not only assess your needs and provide you with advice regarding specific exercises but also help you get started on a fitness program that suits you. In addition, he or she can help you locate other appropriate exercise programs in the community. If you normally use ice or heat for joint or muscle pain, consult with your physical therapist about the proper way of applying these in order to avoid the risks of frostbite or burns.

Consult with your doctor. It is essential that you check with your health professional (e.g., family doctor or physical therapist) if you are starting a new exercise program. Some types of exercise (e.g., for those with certain heart conditions) are not recommended by the American Geriatrics Society (AGS) Panel on Exercise and Osteoarthritis.

Medication. Talk to your physician about any effects your medication use may have on physical activity. Simple modifications may assist you in carrying out your exercise program more appropriately and safely. These changes are especially important if you are taking medications that affect blood pressure or balance. Also, remember that if you are taking any drugs for pain, you should consult with your health professional about the right dosage and timing.

General Guidelines

Variety. This chapter describes activities that are designed to provide many options for exercise and physical activity. Your program of exercise and physical activity should be designed to offer you a variety of activities to encourage regular participation.

Increase intensity slowly. Whenever possible, the exercises and activities should also follow the principles of progressive training. Begin slowly and at a level that is safe and enjoyable, but as you become comfortable and your tolerance increases, raise the level of intensity to produce a training effect. Keep in mind that it will probably *not* be possible for you to participate in vigorous intensity early in the program. Build your capacity slowly.

Adapt to your needs. The exercises and physical activities used should always be adapted, adjusted, or discontinued according to your needs.

Hurt, not harm. Participants with chronic pain may experience soreness and discomfort after exercise. Be aware that there may be some muscle and joint discomfort after an exercise session, but you can keep this soreness to a minimum by carefully planning activities and beginning slowly. Remember that most soreness associated with exercise will not cause harm. *If you feel joint pain during exercise, simply stop.* If this pain persists when you exercise again, it is wise to consult with your physician or physical therapist.

Know your limits. Be cautious, particularly in the early days of your program. Do not overexert yourself, and do not exceed your physical abilities. Learn your own limits.

Talk test. Try to always exercise with a partner. To check on the intensity of exercise, be sure to converse regularly with your partner. You should be working at an intensity level that will make you feel some workload, but you should always be able to respond to questions without gasping or getting breathless. Adjust the intensity of your exercise accordingly.

Breathe regularly. It is also important to make sure that you breathe regularly while you are exercising. Try to concentrate on keeping your breath steady during your exercise session. Do not hold your breath. If you feel it is becoming difficult to maintain normal breathing, or you feel your shoulders shrug up to your ears and find yourself taking short breaths, you are working too hard. Decrease your exercise by slowing down, by taking a short break, or by reducing the intensity of exercise (e.g., lifting less weight).

Monitor-Perceived Exertion. One way to tell whether you are working hard enough is to use what is called a Rating of Perceived Exertion (RPE). This tool (developed by Gunar Borg) rates how hard you feel you are working during your exercise session. The scale ranges from 6 (very, very light) to 20 (maximum exertion). During your exercise session you do not want to exceed a rating of 13 (somewhat hard). Your health professional (e.g., your doctor or a physical therapist) can help you determine what exertion rating is appropriate for you. (At the time of this writing the Rating of Perceived Exertion scale was available on the Internet at *http://www.cdc.gov/nccdphp/dnpa/physical/measuring perceived_exertion.htm.*)

Smooth movements. Keep your movements smooth, gentle, and rhythmical, never sudden, jerky, or too fast. You should not *bounce* while stretching. Understand what body part is the focus of the activity and concentrate on feeling it move.

Know the warning signs. Stop exercising immediately and notify your physician if you notice any of the following:

- Chest pain
- Weakness
- Nausea
- Confusion
- Sudden loss of bowel or bladder control
- Sudden inability to talk (aphasia)

- Shortness of breath
- Light-headedness
- Vertigo (dizziness)
- Blurred vision
- Any new complaint or problem
- Very rapid, slow, or irregular heartbeat/pulse

Avoid exercises and activities that are not recommended for older adults. The following are examples of exercises/activities that are NOT recommended for older adults:

- Exercises/activities that place the head below the heart (can put excessive strain on the heart)

- ◎ Standing, straight-legged toe-touching as a stretching exercise (may cause low back stress)

- ◎ Overhead activities that require extreme positions of the arms and spine and can put undue stress on the cervical spine (neck), shoulders, and back

Realistic goals. For the purposes of this program, physical fitness is defined as the ability to perform all activities of daily living comfortably while still having enough energy to deal with emergencies and not become overly tired. In other words, you are physically fit if you are able to accomplish all of the daily physical tasks that are important to you. When setting your goals, determine realistic activity and fitness levels for a period of time (e.g., 12 weeks). Consult with your doctor or physical therapist to assist in helping you set realistic goals. You may also ask your health care professional to identify programs in the community that offer trained fitness consultants who can assist you in achieving these goals. Some communities have programs designed specifically for older adults with chronic health conditions.

Keep a record. See the end of this chapter for a chart that helps you record your exercise program and progress in performing common activities. Writing down what you did and how it felt will help you determine what works best for you. In addition to this record, you can keep track of how the exercise is affecting various daily functions that you perform. An example of a function scale is also provided. Complete this scale before beginning your exercise and continue with it every week as you do your program (preferably at the same time of the week and same time of day). It is a quick method for seeing how you are progressing relative to the common activities you perform each day. If you are interested in a more detailed evaluation of your function or fitness consult with your health professional. One example of a tool used with older adults is the Functional Fitness Test (FFT), used specifically to evaluate aspects of strength, flexibility, and aerobic performance.

Posture

Posture refers to any position you assume, whether standing, sitting, lying down, or doing any physical activity. It is important to keep good posture as you exercise or when you are resting. If possible, it is better to change positions during your exercise program, rather than sitting or standing one way for long periods of time. Selecting the correct exercise position depends on your abilities and your exercise goals.

Obviously, lying down is the most stable position and is safer than the standing position for performing some of the stretching and strengthening exercises. Sitting is also a fairly stable position and can be used for a variety of fitness exercises. Standing is the least stable position and requires you to have good balance. Standing exercises are very important for improving dynamic activities like walking and stairs. Choose a position that suits your abilities. For example if you are using a walking device, choosing sitting or lying positions to do your strengthening and stretching exercises would be safer and more effective in accomplishing these goals. This is especially important if you are doing your exercises without supervision.

Standing. When standing, keep your earlobe over your shouder and hip as a means of keeping a neutral position. Be sure that your weight is distributed evenly across both feet. A slight bend at the knees helps to stop you from forcing your knees backwards and putting possible strain on knee structures. Refer to Chapter 7 for more specific information on posture while standing. Try to keep this position during standing exercises. If you can't keep good posture while doing these exercises, you should take a break and then resume exercising. Focusing on good standing posture will strengthen the trunk muscles and help you perform other physical activties that occur in standing positions.

Sitting. Sitting is a good exercise position for people who find that they have increased joint pain when standing or for those who have difficulty with balance. In general, you should not slouch. However, not everyone has the ability to easily sit in the *ideal* position described above. If you have difficulty sitting, choose another position to carry out your exercises. If your chair is less than

74

ideal, you may choose to use towels to support the back (as demonstrated in the picture).

Whether you use a chair for sitting (see Chapter 7) or for exercise, it should be high enough that your feet are flat on the ground. Your chair should also allow you to sit with your weight equally distributed through both buttocks. Try exercising in a chair without a back. This will strengthen your tummy and back by making you work the muscles harder. On the other hand, if you need more back support, use a chair with arms and a back. Obviously, if you have a more supportive chair it will limit the amount of movement you can carry out.

If you sit for extended periods of time on a regular basis (e.g., half an hour or more), get up and/or stretch every 20 to 30 minutes. Refer to Chapter 7 for more specific information on posture while sitting.

Lying on your back and on yourside. If you spend a great deal of time lying in bed, it is important to support the head, neck, spine, arms, and legs in more *neutral* positions. The photographs below emphasize these *neutral* positions. In the first figure maximum comfort can be achieved when the knees are slightly bent and a pillow is placed under the whole length of the leg. This position takes some stress off the low back as well as the knees. Placing the pillow under the thigh and lower leg keeps it from putting excessive pressure on the sensitive structures under the knee.

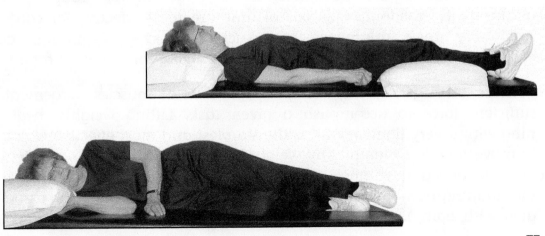

Chapter Six | *The Role of Exercise in Seniors' Lives*

You may find that lying on your side is most comfortable and offers good support. Try experimenting to find which size pillow gives the best support to your head, neck, and shoulders.

For most people it is difficult to stay in one position for long periods of time. Changing posture often is a good way to stay comfortable. Again, whenever possible, keep your body in *neutral* positions. Try putting a long *body pillow* in front of you as you lie on your side. Rest your top arm and top leg on this pillow (not shown in the picture) and see if it makes you more comfortable.

Components of Fitness

If you were asked to define the essential components of an exercise program, what would you include? Strength training? Cardiovascular fitness? Becoming more flexible? It is likely that the elements you include in your program will be based on your background and present health needs. Generally speaking, physical fitness includes six components.

- Cardiorespiratory fitness
- Muscle endurance
- Flexibility
- Muscle strength
- Range of motion (movement)
- Body composition

A complete program includes activities designed to enhance all six. Each one is explained below.

Cardiorespiratory fitness is the capacity of the heart, lungs, and circulatory system to deliver oxygenated blood throughout the body. Activities that require movement of the large muscle groups, such as the thighs, for longer periods of time are most effective for cardio respiratory fitness training. Exercises such as walking, swimming, and cycling are among the most effective for improving this aspect of fitness.

Muscle strength is the ability of the skeletal muscles to generate sufficient force to accomplish a given task. Lifting weights, beginning with a very light weight, is the simplest and most effective way to improve muscle strength. Any weight-lifting or weight-bearing activity has the added advantage of loading the skeleton and assisting in maintaining bone density (i.e., reducing the bone loss usually associated with aging). Increasing your muscle strength may help provide additional support for weakened joints. Normally, strengthening involves fewer repetitions of an exercise. As you improve your strength, you may do more than one set of repetitions.

Muscle endurance is the ability of the skeletal muscles to generate movement over a long period of time. To gain muscle endurance, you must increase the number of repetitions that you do for your strengthening exercise (i.e., more than 12 repetitions).

Range of motion (movement) refers to the normal amount that the joints can move. This element is crucial for independent living. A simple task such as combing the hair on the back of your head requires significant shoulder, elbow, wrist, and finger movements. Joints have different directions and different levels of movement. For example, the knee only straightens and bends, while the hip moves out and in, moves forward and back, and also turns in and out. As you age, the amount of movement in the joints normally decreases. This loss can, however, be reduced with exercise. A range of motion exercise allows you to focus on moving a particular joint. For example, to improve the mobility of your elbow, you would first flex it (i.e., bend your elbow so that your hand comes to your shoulder) and then extend it (i.e., straighten your elbow). The emphasis in these exercises is on moving the joint through positions that are used during common functions and activities.

Everything surrounding the joint, including muscles, tendons, joint capsules, and bony structures, is involved in range of motion exercises, which are typically performed without resistance and can be done prior to any form of exercise. Range of motion movements may be used as a warm-up for a specific joint or area of the body. Also, it is important to take the joints through their complete motions on a regular basis in order to prevent stiffness and loss of easy movement.

Flexibility is about stretching. Flexibility and range of motion exercises are somewhat different from one another. The purpose of flexibility is to make certain the muscles around the joints do not become shortened. Stretching exercises may help to prevent your muscles from shortening and tightening, which may increase your pain. Stretching is best done after range of motion exercises, which will have increased circulation and required movement of other joint structures (bone, joint capsule, and ligaments). Also, stretching seems to be easier to perform when the body is warmer, so it is often better to do stretching exercises after you get warmed up a bit or after you have had a warm bath or shower.

Body composition, as a component of fitness, relates primarily to the percentage of body mass made up of fat. The body is a combination of bone, muscle, fat, and a variety of other tissues (e.g., nerves, blood). A high amount of body fat is a tremendous burden for the cardiorespiratory and muscle/bone systems and makes the goal of overall fitness difficult to attain. Two important contributors to the percentage of body fat are nutrition (i.e., what you eat) and physical activity/exercise. All physical activity helps burn calories, and regular physical activity is critical to maintaining proper body weight. If exercise or the performance of physical activities is painful or uncomfortable, seek professional advice to help you find options for increasing physical activity and alternative exercise programs.

Outline of a General Exercise Program

Below, we provide an outline for a general exercise program followed by an explanation of each of the components and finally pictures describing some of the exercises. As always, the exercises and activities that follow should be adapted to fit your needs. The exercises have been grouped in sections, beginning with suggestions for warming up.

Depending on your present level of function and any health concerns you may have, the frequency, intensity, and duration of each of these components will need to be tailored to suit you. Speak to your health professional about what exercises you should be doing, how often, and at what level of difficulty. The examples below are arranged starting with easier options and moving on to ones that are more difficult. Begin with activities seated in a chair and progress to a standing position when appropriate. The end of the chapter also has some suggestions of alternative activities you may enjoy.

Warm-Up Exercises (5 to 10 Minutes)

Number of Repetitions: Start out performing exercises 5 to 10 times and build as you progress.

Options:

- ⊚ Using arm muscles perform biceps curls (seated OR standing) — see pg. 81 and pg. 82
- ⊚ Marching (seated OR standing) — see pg. 81 and pg. 82
- ⊚ Marching (seated OR standing with some arm activity) — see pg. 81 and pg. 82
- ⊚ Shoulder rolls — see pg. 82
- ⊚ Ankle/foot rotation — see pg. 83

Aerobic Exercises (15 to 20 Minutes)

Duration: Start with 5 minutes and gradually build up your tolerance.

Options:

- ⊚ Marching (seated) — see pg. 84
- ⊚ Walking inside or outside — see pg. 84
- ⊚ Climbing stairs — see pg. 84

Strengthening Exercises

Note: *You can do these exercises after your warm-up either after or instead of a brief aerobic workout. Remember that the number of repetitions depends on your goals and should slowly progress. Pick those exercises that are important for your goals.*

Options:

- ⊚ Mini-squat (leg strength) — see pg. 86
  OR full-chair squat — see pg. 87 OR assisted
  chair squat (using arms) — pg. 87

  (**Note:** *If you have low back problems, it is not recommended that you do this exercise repeatedly.*)

- ⊚ Elbow extensions — see pg. 88
- ⊚ Elbow flexion (biceps curls) — see pg. 89
- ⊚ Abdominal squeeze with a backward lean — see pg. 89

- ◎ Wrist curls (seated) — see pg. 90
- ◎ Wrist extensions (seated) — see pg. 90
- ◎ Ball squeeze — see pg. 91
- ◎ Web squeeze — see pg. 91
- ◎ Shoulder squeeze — see pg. 91
- ◎ Wall pushups — see pg. 92

Flexibility Exercises

Note: You can do flexibility exercises after your warm-up in place of an aerobic program, or you can add a gentle stretching session following your aerobic exercise.

Options:
- ◎ Chest stretch (seated OR standing) — see pg. 93
- ◎ Shoulder and upper back stretch — see pg. 93
- ◎ Reach-up stretch (seated) — see pg. 94
- ◎ Forearm/wrist flexor stretch (seated) – see pg. 94
- ◎ Forearm/wrist extensor stretch (seated) — see pg. 95
- ◎ Hamstring stretch (seated) — see pg. 95
- ◎ Ankle stretch, toe forward (seated) — see pg. 96
- ◎ Ankle stretch, calf stretch (seated) — see pg. 96

Cool-Down Exercises (5 to 10 Minutes)
Options:
- ◎ Marching (seated OR standing)—see pg. 97

Warm-Up Activities

When you exercise, do you jump right in or do you take some time to warm up? Regardless of age, a good warm-up is very important before exercise. As the word implies, warm-up activities are designed to heat the muscles, increase blood flow to the extremities, and get the body ready for exercise. Proper warm-up and stretching exercises will allow for increased ease of movement and will help prevent injuries. Warm-up exercises may benefit individuals with chronic pain by helping to reduce muscle stiffness and improve ease of movement. Generally, 5 to 10 minutes should be spent on warm-up activities.

Biceps Curls (Seated) – Easy

Move your arms from the elbows, bending your forearms up toward your upper arms.

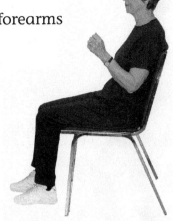

Marching (Seated) – Easy

Lift your feet off the floor (moving from your hips) as if you are walking in place.

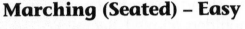

Note: *Be aware that this may be difficult if you have poor hip or spine movement.*

Marching with Biceps Curl (Seated) – More Advanced

To make seated marching more challenging, try adding some arm movement by lifting the opposite arm to accompany the leg motion. Remember to begin slowly to get the muscles warm.

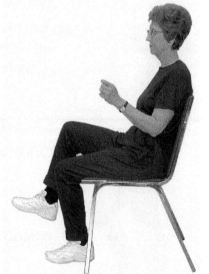

If you have difficulty with hip movements you can gently lift the feet off the floor by straightening the knees and pulling the toes up. This will encourage movement at the knees and ankles involving the surrounding muscle, bones, and other tissues.

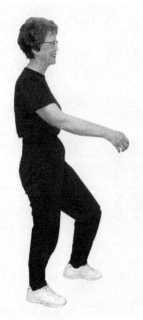

Marching on the Spot (Standing) – Easier

If you feel comfortable, marching can also be done from a standing position. Remember to watch your posture—stand up straight and keep your shoulders relaxed. Begin by holding onto a chair. In time, you may be able to complete this exercise unsupported.

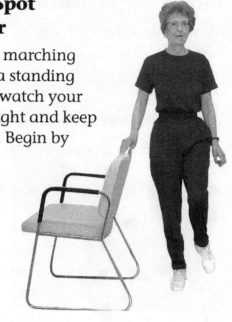

Marching Biceps Curl (Standing) – More Advanced

To make marching on the spot more difficult, add an arm motion, bending your elbow and bringing your forearm to your upper arm (biceps curl).

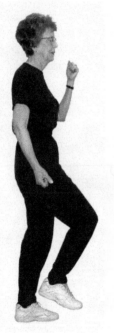

Shoulder Rolls (Seated or Standing)

Once your body is warm, you want to get the joints moving. Begin by slowly and gently rolling your shoulders backward and forward a few times. Remember to keep your head and neck in a neutral position.

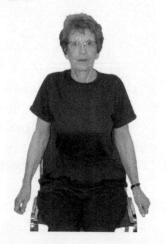
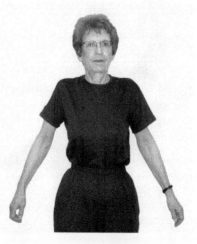

Ankle/Foot Rotation (Seated)

To warm up the ankle joints, gently rotate them one at a time in a clockwise and then counter-clockwise direction. Again, make sure the movements are slow and controlled.

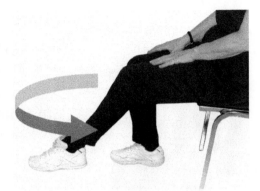

Aerobic Activities

Now that you're warmed up, you may choose to begin with some aerobic exercises. Activities that are continuous and use large muscle groups are considered to be aerobic exercise. The American Geriatrics Society has made several recommendations that we describe in this section. First, they suggest that you select a variety of aerobic exercise options. A variety of exercises will reduce the likelihood of overusing specific joints while preventing you from becoming bored with your exercise program. Examples include bicycling, swimming, using treadmills and rowing machines, and engaging in other low-impact activities such as walking or dancing. Keep in mind that certain daily activities (e.g., yard work, playing a sport, or walking to the store) are also practical forms of aerobic exercise! For those who experience discomfort with load-bearing exercises, aquatic activities may be preferable because they offer buoyant support.

A goal of 20 to 30 minutes per day is optimal for individuals who are just beginning an exercise program. For some individuals, this goal may not be possible for medical or functional reasons. Tailor this goal to suit your abilities. Where necessary, aerobic activities can be accumulated in shorter 5- or 10-minute intervals. Remember that aerobic activities do not have to be strenuous. If you are just beginning an exercise program, you should try to exercise at least three days per week but no more than four days per week. Older adults who begin a fitness program by exercising 5 or more times per week may place themselves at increased risk for injury. This does not apply to individuals who are already active in an exercise program. *Make sure that the progression of your aerobic training is gradual to allow time for your body to adapt (i.e., 2 to 3 months).* A variety of aerobic exercises are presented below that do not require any special equipment. See which ones work for you!

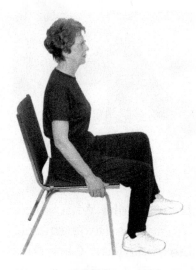

Marching (Seated)

Note: *This exercise requires good hip and spine mobility and stability.*

Alternately lift your feet off the floor as if you are walking in place. If you completed this as part of your warm-up, try lifting your knees a little higher or marching a bit more quickly to make it more challenging. Remember to use the *talk test* (described earlier in this chapter) to ensure that you are not working too hard.

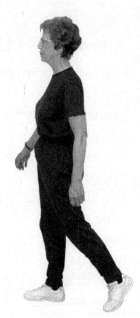

Walking Inside

If you feel comfortable walking, find a clear, safe path inside to go for a stroll. As with the marching activities described above, use the talk test to ensure you are exercising within recommended limits. Remember to wear appropriate footwear.

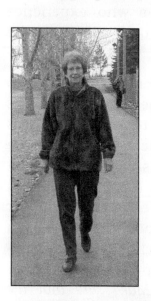

Walking Outside

If you feel comfortable walking outside, find a clear, safe path to use. As above, use the talk test to ensure that you are exercising within recommended limits.

Climbing Stairs

Stair climbing is a more challenging activity, but it can be used as part of your aerobic exercise routine.

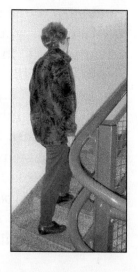

Start slowly and build up. Whenever possible, make sure that you use stairs that have handrails for additional support and safety.

Strengthening Activities

These days, it is widely recognized that strengthening activities are beneficial for older adults. The goal in these training programs is to maintain muscle strength and endurance. If you choose to try some of the strengthening activities described in this section, consider the guidelines (supplemented with recommendations from the American Geriatrics Society) that are provided below.

It is important to use slow, continuous movement through a full range of motion wherever possible. You should feel some tension in the muscles as part of your exercise routines and physical activity. However, in general you should avoid exercising until you are at the point of muscle fatigue.

Begin by attempting to repeat the exercise several times (e.g., one set of four to six repetitions). If you do not feel tired, try adding a few more repetitions until the muscles feel tired. If you are able to complete 15 repetitions easily, it is time to move to a more challenging intensity of exercise and reduce the number of times the exercise is repeated. Usually increasing intensity means that you provide some resistance to the movement using weights or other types of resistance training equipment. Remember that if you keep the repetitions lower, you work more on muscle strength. Be sure that breathing is not restricted— do not hold your breath when lifting weights. You may need to modify your strengthening exercises to accommodate functional limitations (e.g., pain or inflamed joints).

Strengthening exercises are most effective when performed three times per week with a day's rest in between. Allow for a gradual progression in any resistance exercises. Remember to work at your own pace, and listen to your body. Talk to your health professional about how to fit these exercises with your aerobic exercise program to ensure you gain the benefits without overdoing it! For some individuals, it may be necessary to begin by lifting lighter weights (e.g., bean bags, soup cans) and progress to other equipment. For others, lifting weights might not be possible.

Mini-Squat

Note: *Although this exercise strengthens the muscles of your upper legs, it is not recommended for individuals with low back problems.*

Stand approximately six inches in front of your chair with your feet shoulder width apart. Use another chair or arrange yourself in front of a stable object such as a counter-top. Maintain your posture, keeping your back straight as you lower yourself slowly as if you are going to sit down. Go down only as far as you feel comfortable. Reverse direction to return to an upright position of standing. This exercise uses the large muscles of the upper leg. Remember to breathe as you do this activity. Do not hold your breath. Again, if you have lower back problems, it would not be recommended to do this exercise repeatedly. You also need good ankle movement to perform this exercise effectively.

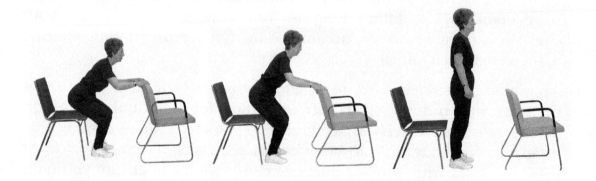

Note: *These exercises are good from a functional standpoint (e.g., sitting down in a chair and getting up from a chair). If you wish to increase your repetitions, consider doing the squats while leaning against a wall (i.e., wall squats) because your back will be better aligned.*

A few options of varying difficulty for the squat exercise are shown below.

Full Chair Squat – Advanced

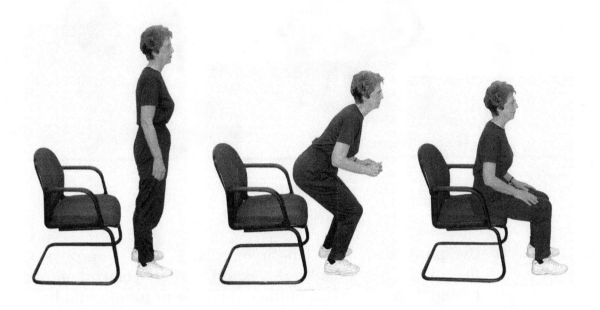

Assisted Chair Squat (Using Arms)

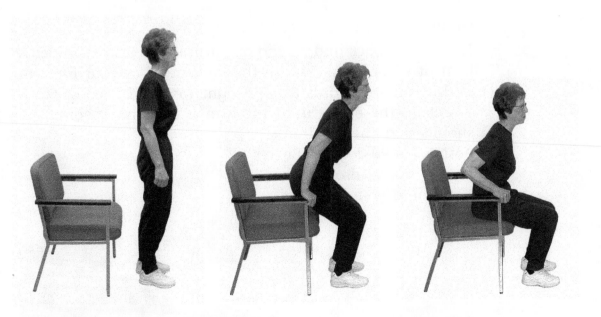

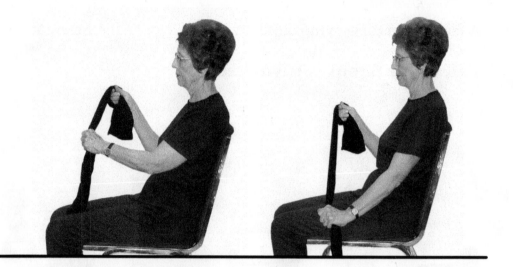

Elbow Extensions

Option 1:

⊚ Use pantyhose or a length of tubing. Ask your physio-therapist or other health professional where you can obtain tubing. Grasp one end of the pantyhose or tubing and hold that arm in a stable position. Take hold of the other end and pull it away until your arm is straight. Release slowly and repeat. Watch that the tubing is secure so it does not snap back into your body.

Option 2:

⊚ Lie on your back and extend one arm up so your shoulder is bent at 90 degrees. Control the movement of your forearm and hand downwards using a light weight if needed. Slowly extend the elbow until the arm is straight, keeping the shoulder in the original position of 90 degrees. Be careful not to drop your hand onto your head or face.

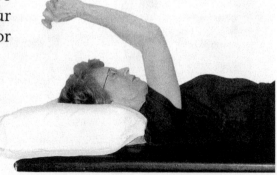

Elbow Flexion – Biceps Curl

In a seated position, with a light weight if needed, begin with one forearm relaxed in your lap and the upper arm straight down by the side of your body. Bend the elbow up as far as you are able while keeping the upper arm still. Slowly relax the arm back down to your lap and repeat.

Abdominal Squeeze with a Backward Lean (Seated)

Sit slightly forward in a chair, remembering to maintain good posture. Ensure that your seat has good contact with the chair so you do not slip off the chair. Breathe out as you lean backward slightly without letting your back touch the chair. Lean back only as far as you feel comfortable while still being able to bring yourself back to an upright position. This exercise also works the muscles in the front of your neck, so if you have neck problems it might not be recommended. Make sure the chair is stable so that it does not tip.

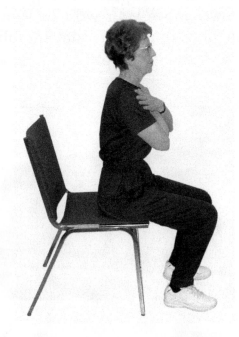 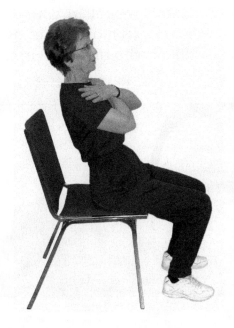

Wrist Curls (Seated)

Note: If you do not have weights you can use household items such as a can of soup or a bag of rice.

With your forearm resting on the arm of a chair, palm facing up, hold a small weight in your hand. Slowly move your wrist as shown below. Repeat as many times as you are able, and do the same number of repetitions with the other arm.

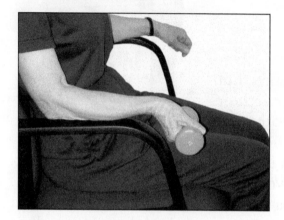 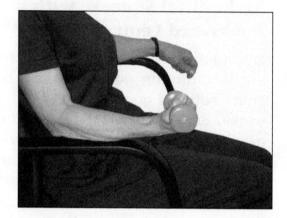

Wrist Extensions (Seated)

With your forearm resting on the arm of a chair, palm facing down, hold a small weight in your hand. Slowly move your wrist as shown below. Repeat as many times as you are able, and do the same number of repetitions with the other arm.

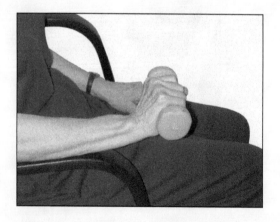 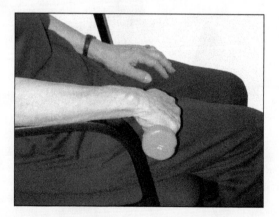

Ball Squeeze (Seated)

Holding a rolled-up sock or a ball in your hand, gently squeeze, hold for a few seconds, and then release. Repeat until the muscles in your forearms feel tired.

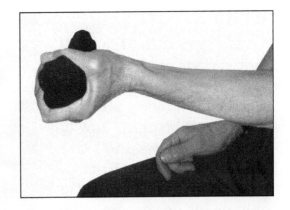

Web Squeeze (Seated)

As an alternative to the ball squeeze, you may wish to use a web or other grip-strengthening tool. As shown below, squeeze gently, hold for a few seconds, and then release. Repeat until the muscles in your forearms feel tired.

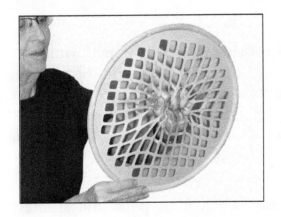

If you are interested in more specific exercises for the management of hand pain, please consult with a physical or occupational therapist.

Shoulder Blade Squeeze (Seated and Standing)

Lift your elbows out to the side. Breathe out as you draw your elbows back and squeeze your shoulder blades together. Hold for a few seconds and then relax.

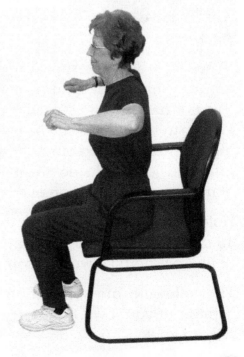

Wall Pushup

Find a space on the wall that is clear of obstructions. Stand six inches away and place your hands against it, shoulder width apart. Slowly bend your elbows and lower your chest to the wall, keeping your back straight. Go only as far as you are able. When you are ready, slowly extend your elbows and push yourself away from the wall.

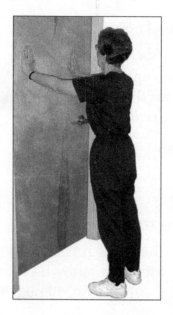
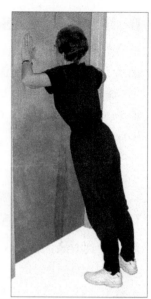

Stretching Activities

Once you have warmed up your muscles and joints, performing a program of light stretching will assist in improving range of motion. Stretching is important, given that many seniors with chronic pain problems experience limitations in their range of motion. We suggest following the guidelines for stretching that we describe in this section, which have been supplemented with recommendations from the American Geriatrics Society.

If possible, do your stretching exercises when your pain and stiffness are at a minimum, and be sure to take time to relax before you start. It is not necessary to stretch to the full range of motion to gain benefit. When stretching, *less can be better.* You may need to modify your stretching exercises to accommodate functional limitations (e.g., pain or inflamed joints). To do so, it might be necessary to reduce the range of motion or the duration of the stretch.

Hold a stretch (i.e., feel some tension in the muscle) for up to a count of 15 or as tolerated. Do *not* bounce. Stretching exercises can be performed daily and should always accompany aerobic or strengthening exercises.

The following are some stretching activities you can perform in the comfort of your own home. Try each to see which ones are possible and helpful for you.

Chest Stretch (Seated or Standing)

In a seated position, keeping the spine erect as shown, move your arms backwards to feel a stretch in the chest region. By squeezing your shoulder blades together at the same time you will help to extend your shoulders. A more advanced standing stretch can be accomplished by clasping your hands behind your back. This exercise requires very good movement of the shoulder; if you have shoulder problems it may create discomfort, and so it may not be advised. Hold the position for up to 15 seconds and watch that you do not arch your back.

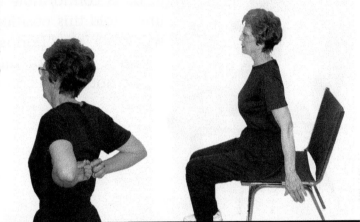

Shoulder and Upper Back Stretch (Seated or Standing)

Begin with your arms stretched comfortably out to the side. Gently bring them in front of your body and alternate right over left and left over right. Make your movements large, smooth and controlled.

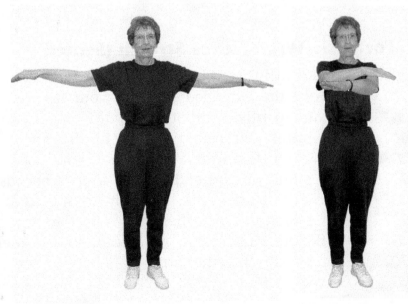

Chapter Six | *The Role of Exercise in Seniors' Lives*

Reach-Up Stretch (Seated or Standing)

Note: This exercise is easier to do if you are lying on your back with your knees bent up. If you can't get down onto the floor, lying on your couch is fine.

Sit or stand, making certain to maintain good posture. Bring your arms up over your head as high as is comfortable and gently reach for the ceiling. Hold this position for a few seconds, then slowly lower your hands to your sides. Keep your back flat if at all possible (otherwise you do not stretch the muscles as effectively).

Forearm/Wrist Flexor Stretch (Seated)

Extend one arm in front of you with the palm facing away. Take the extended hand in your free hand and gently bend it backward toward you until you feel a stretch in the front of your forearm. Watch that you do not pull on the ends of the fingers because the purpose is primarily to stretch the forearm/wrist flexors, not the finger flexors. Hold for up to 15 seconds, and then repeat with the other arm.

94

Forearm/Wrist Extensor Stretch (Seated)

With your arm extended straight ahead and your palm facing toward you, take hold just above the knuckles with your free hand and gently pull your wrist and fingers toward you until you feel a stretch in the back of your forearm. Again, this exercise is primarily meant to stretch the forearm/wrist extensor muscles. Hold for up to 15 seconds, and then repeat with the other arm.

Hamstring Stretch (Seated)

Sit forward in your chair with one leg extended in front of you, heel on the floor and knee straight. Maintain good posture while bending forward from the hip. Think about pressing your chest forward. Lean far enough so that you feel a stretch in the back of the outstretched leg. Do not lock your knee but keep it comfortably straight. Hold for up to 15 seconds and repeat with the other leg. Watch that you are stretching the back of your leg and not your back!

Ankle Stretch – Toe Pointed Forward (Seated)

In a seated position, gently point your toe until you feel a stretch in the front of your lower leg (your shin). Hold for up to 15 seconds and then repeat with the other leg. This exercise can be done with the knee straight or with it bent. Different muscles are stretched with each knee position.

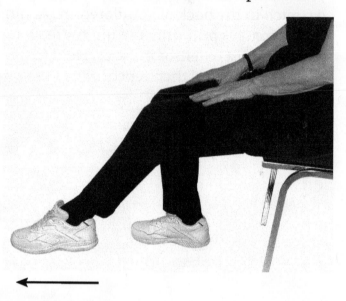

Ankle Stretch – Calf Stretch (Seated)

In a seated position, gently draw your toe toward your shin until you feel a stretch in the back of your lower leg (calf). Hold for up to 15 seconds and then repeat on the other leg.

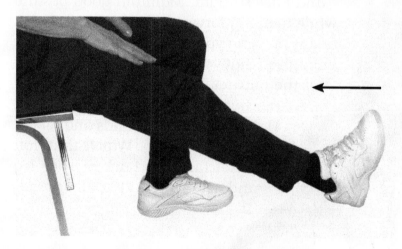

Cool-Down Activities

Many people who exercise regularly warm up at the beginning but fail to cool down at the end. This is unfortunate, because cool-down activities help reduce discomfort and muscle stiffness that may be felt the next day. It is recommended that at the end of any aerobic activity you cool down using exercises such as the ones you performed for your warm-up. A good cool-down activity is marching in a seated or standing position for 5 minutes.

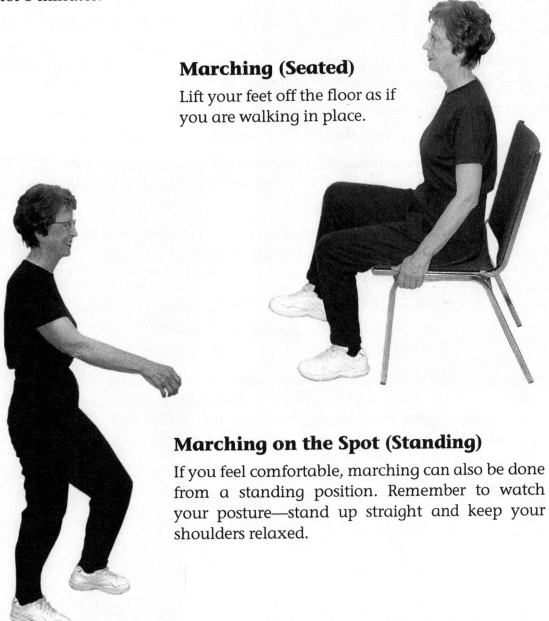

Marching (Seated)

Lift your feet off the floor as if you are walking in place.

Marching on the Spot (Standing)

If you feel comfortable, marching can also be done from a standing position. Remember to watch your posture—stand up straight and keep your shoulders relaxed.

Setting Goals and Changing Them to Suit Your Needs

Now that you have reviewed the outline of a general exercise program (i.e., the warm-up, aerobic activities, strengthening activities, stretching activities, cool-down activities), you are ready to put your program into action! When you determine how much time to spend on each of the components of exercise, remember to match these to your specific goals. In general, improving your physical activity will also improve your function and reduce pain. Although it is suggested that older adults attempt to exercise for 30 minutes almost every day, this goal may not be appropriate for you. Select your activities and the amount of time you exercise according to your abilities.

- If you have poor joint mobility you may want to focus primarily on the warm-up and flexibility components.

- For individuals who have muscle weakness it may be most appropriate to do the warm-up and strengthening components.

- If your goal is to improve general activity levels and fitness, you should focus on the warm-up, aerobic, and cool-down components.

- If you want to achieve all of these benefits, work on all aspects of the fitness program. Consider the overall amount of exercise as you do not want to overdo it!

Pick what works best for you. The most important issue is to select an exercise or physical activity program that allows you to keep doing it regularly. Always start slowly, working for a few minutes and then progressing as you are able to tolerate more exercise.

The following are examples of ways to change your exercise program as you progress:

For Stretching:

- ◎ Hold the position a little longer (an extra 5 to 10 seconds).

- ◎ Go a little farther into the range of movement.

- ◎ Do a few more repetitions (start with one or two and move to three or four).

For Strengthening:

- ◎ Lift a heavier weight or increase resistance with tubing.

- ◎ Move through more range of movement with the weight.

- ◎ Keep a low number of repetitions with a heavier weight.

For Aerobics:

- ◎ Exercise for a longer period of time.

- ◎ Exercise daily.

- ◎ Do more repetitions of an exercise.

Important Things to Watch For

1. Pain should not increase as you exercise.

2. You might feel stiff at the beginning of your program, but this should improve as you move through the exercises.

3. You should have good control during the exercise so that you don't force a joint or body part into an unsafe position. Remember to maintain good posture while performing the exercises — using a mirror is often helpful in checking your body position.

4. If pain comes on following the exercise, you have possibly done too much. You may need advice as to what you should and should not do.

5. If your joint or muscle area becomes red or hot after you exercise, you may have overdone it. Ask a health professional how to modify your program.

6. Remember that there are two excellent ways to make sure you are not working too hard: the talk test and monitoring your heart rate.

7. Remember not to hold your breath.

8. If you feel exhausted or are unable to sleep at night after exercising, you could be doing too much. Ask for advice from you physician or physical therapist.

9. You should not have difficulty doing any of your other daily activities after exercising. If you do, you have done too much. In most cases, people find that function improves once they get going on an exercise program.

10. You should NOT increase your pain medication because of exercises unless your physician advises it. Again, increased pain may be a sign of overdoing your exercises or not doing them properly.

Summary

The physical and psychological benefits of regular exercise far outweigh the costs when it comes to managing chronic pain. Working with your health professional, you can effectively integrate an exercise program into your chronic pain management. We hope this chapter has either confirmed your commitment to maintaining your physical health through regular exercise or led you to begin an appropriate exercise program. In addition, we hope that you have learned about the essential components of a sound exercise program and the importance of setting realistic and flexible goals. If you are just beginning an exercise program, remember that it may be difficult to *get in the groove* at first. However, if you stick with it, exercise will become a part of your regular routine. The ultimate goals are to more effectively manage your chronic pain and enjoy the on-going rewards of having a higher level of physical fitness. Be sure to refer back to the contents of this chapter as you begin or modify your exercise activities.

Other Physical Activity Program Options

There are many other forms of physical training and exercise that can be included or modified for use in programs by older adults. Two excellent options include yoga and T'ai Chi. Both can be modified to meet the needs of participants with different levels of exercise tolerance. It is best to perform these activities in a class with a certified instructor. Before your class begins, let the instructor know if you have any special conditions or problem areas so that he or she can help you to modify the exercises or suggest other options. Brief descriptions of these two physical activity programs follow.

Yoga

Yoga originated in India thousands of years ago. It encompasses a holistic approach to physical and mental health. There are many different kinds of yoga. *Hatha yoga* is the physical yoga that helps you gain control over your body through various postures and breathing exercises. The physical benefits derived from yoga (increased flexibility, strength, power, and stamina) may help some older adults cope with chronic pain more effectively. For example, pain that is related to stiff, contracted muscles and joints may be alleviated through exercises.

The practice of yoga also serves to promote mental health and the adoption of a balanced, flexible approach to life. A more easy-going attitude is a definite asset among older adults with chronic pain, given that it is sometimes necessary to accommodate oneself to changing levels of functioning.

The distinguishing characteristics of yoga make it a beneficial system of movement for older adults. These characteristics include body alignment; muscular balance; spinal extension and trunk alignment; and slow, conscious movement combined with breathing techniques.

T'ai Chi

T'ai Chi Chuan, or T'ai Chi as it is commonly known, is first and foremost a martial art, but is used in Western cultures for health purposes. T'aiChi is a form of meditation, a dance, and a way of life. While beneficial for all ages, the traditional forms of T'ai Chi are difficult to learn. There are, however, modified versions and individual T'ai Chi movements that may be done to prepare for the more elaborate forms.

Finding an enjoyable exercise that suits your lifestyle, interests, and physical abilities is most important. Both yoga and T'ai Chi are becoming increasingly popular with older adults and offer a variety of benefits specifically related to improved strength, flexibility, coordination, and balance. It is very important that you do some research when selecting a program to ensure that you are working with an individual who has qualifications and understands the special needs of older adults. In addition, there are valuable resources such as books, videos, CDs, and DVDs that may be helpful so you can perform these exercises in your home. Consult with community organizations as well as health professionals in finding good resources that are right for you.

Exercise Chart

This chart is designed to help you develop good exercise habits. Use it to monitor your progress. Feel free to make copies of this page for your personal use.

Date (m/d/y)	Warm-up Exercises + Time	Done?	Aerobic Exercises + Time	Done?	Strengthening Exercises + Time	Done?	Cool-down Exercises + Time	Done?	Stretching Exercises + Time	Done?
		Y N		Y N		Y N		Y N		Y N
		Y N		Y N		Y N		Y N		Y N
		Y N		Y N		Y N		Y N		Y N
		Y N		Y N		Y N		Y N		Y N
		Y N		Y N		Y N		Y N		Y N
		Y N		Y N		Y N		Y N		Y N
		Y N		Y N		Y N		Y N		Y N
		Y N		Y N		Y N		Y N		Y N
		Y N		Y N		Y N		Y N		Y N
		Y N		Y N		Y N		Y N		Y N

Chapter Six | *The Role of Exercise in Seniors' Lives*

Function Scale

These questions will help you rate your ability to carry out common activities. In addition to the few examples that are given, please add other activities that you do daily. You may photocopy this questionnaire for your personal use. Complete the questionnaire before you start doing an exercise program, and then go back and answer the questions once every four weeks. This will help you review the benefits of your exercise program.

Date: _____ Time: _____

Check only those questions that are appropriate to your activities:

	Unable to do	Able to do with significant difficulty	Able to do with moderate difficulty	Able to do with some difficulty	Able to do with no difficulty
1. Sleeping					
2. Sitting (for 10 minutes or longer)					
3. Standing (for 10 minutes or longer)					
4.					
5.					
6					
7.					
8.					
9.					
10.					
11.					
12.					
13.					
14.					

NANCY K. TURNER, MSC
ELIZABETH L. HARRISON, PHD, DPT
ROBERT McCULLOCH, PHD
RONALD R. MARTIN, PHD, RD PSYCH.

CHAPTER SEVEN

Living in More Comfort: Maximizing Function and Energy

Do you consistently lift things safely? Is your home set up to help you manage your pain in the most effective way? You might find that small adjustments to your home and the way that you do everyday activities (e.g., lifting) can make a big difference in helping you handle your ongoing pain. This chapter includes some simple recommendations that you may want to consider while performing common activities of daily living.

For all tasks, make sure that you have proper lighting and appropriate temperature and ventilation, and avoid remaining in noisy environments for extended periods of time. All of these factors (e.g., poor lighting and ventilation) contribute to stress levels and excessive muscle activity, which can lead to fatigue and increased pain. Try to conserve energy, avoid overexerting your muscles, and use safe and effective body positions. If you do a bit of planning, you can accomplish these goals and reduce pain!

To begin with, let's look at different aspects of your home and your daily life that might be targets for change. As you read through each section, consider your own situation (how you do these different activities, or how your home is arranged). See if there are any changes that can be made to assist you in maximizing function while reducing or avoiding pain.

105

Resting/Sleeping

You will feel better if you get proper rest. In addition to getting enough rest at night, some individuals may find it helpful to have a nap during the day, although this depends on the individual and his or her lifestyle. Remember that for some individuals, sleeping during the day-time may interfere with getting good sleep at night.

No single mattress or bed design is superior. Choose your sleeping surface and pillows according to what you find provides some support and yet still allows you the ability to move around in bed. Generally, it is a good idea to try to keep your spine and limbs in neutral positions (see the photograph below) instead of putting yourself in extreme positions. Placing a pillow between your knees can be helpful. Sleep patterns have an influence on pain management. If you have difficulty sleeping, discuss this problem with your health professional. There may be ways to improve your sleep.

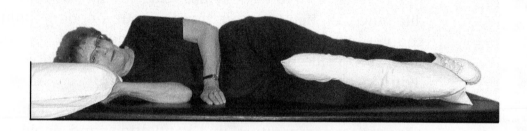

Dressing

Dressing requires good manual dexterity of the hands and fingers. If you have pain in these joints, consider choosing clothes that do not have difficult buttons or clasps. Front-opening tops and shirts tend to be easier to put on than pullovers, especially if you have limited shoulder movement. Zipper rings can also be attached to jackets and sweaters to help alleviate pain in your finger joints. Brassieres that clasp in the front are easier to wear than those with back clasps. Tighter fitting clothing tends to be more difficult to get on and off and can limit circulation. Tight pants can be especially problematic if you have limited movement in the hips or knees. If you wear socks that come up to the knee, make sure that the elastic is not too tight because it can also limit circulation.

Women often prefer support hose instead of socks; however, the hose should have a comfortable waistband so the top does not dig into the waist.

Footwear should be chosen for comfort and support. Stay away from high heels or shoes with little support. In addition, choose shoes with good treads to avoid slipping. On the other hand, soles that are too sticky sometimes lead to tripping. So, think about good tread when selecting your footwear. If you have foot problems, it is wise to wear supportive shoes around the house. If you have difficulty tying laces or putting your shoes on, you can find very supportive slip-on loafers, or use a long-handled shoehorn.

Carrying out Basic Hygiene in the Bathroom

In order to maximize safety and improve independence, it is important to consider the setup of the bathroom. If you have good lighting around the mirror, you will not have to strain to see your reflection. To minimize the risk of slipping or falling, avoid having loose rugs or water on the floor as these can lead to accidents. Grab-bars can be installed so that you have appropriate support for bathing, showering, and getting on and off the toilet. It is essential that grab-bars be installed appropriately for safety and your specific needs. Towel bars are not meant to be used as grab-bars—they will pull away from the wall.

If you have pain, or if you have poor movement or weakness in your legs, installing a raised toilet seat can be very helpful. Reducing the amount of forward bending requires less movement in all joints, especially in your back and legs. Think about where your toilet paper holder is located; make sure you don't have to turn or strain to reach it.

Although showering also requires less movement in the legs and spine, some people find it tiring to stand for a length of time. If you have a grab-bar in the shower, make sure it is installed properly. If you are looking for a new shower, consider one that has a seat. Make sure the shower seat is the right height and has a finish that is not slippery.

If you prefer bathing, there are bath benches that can be added to the tub. Getting down into a bathtub requires a good deal of movement and strength in the legs, arms, and spine. Simple modifications to your bathtub (e.g., a bath seat, grab-bars) can make bathing enjoyable instead of a strenuous, painful experience.

An occupational therapist can visit your home and provide practical suggestions and advice on assistive devices or equipment. In addition, there are stores that deal specifically with selling and installing bathroom furniture and fixtures. Consider this an important investment for making bathing a pleasant experience and for preventing falls and slips.

Kitchen Setup

Safety and comfort in the kitchen can easily be improved. For example, place heavier items in locations where you can safely lift them. Put common household items in places that limit the amount you have to reach, and avoid standing on objects in the kitchen (e.g., chairs, stools) as these positions can lead to falls. Here are some simple suggestions for setting up your kitchen:

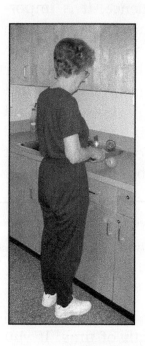

- Keep floors clean to avoid slipping.
- Remove loose rugs.
- Remove clutter along commonly traveled paths.
- Counter height should be at elbow level.

Changing the height of counters is often not possible, but if you do more labor-intensive cooking, perhaps sitting at a table would be beneficial.

Many kitchen utensils require fine movements of the fingers and hands. If you have trouble gripping objects, there are devices available to make using utensils much easier (see the photographs on page 109). Again, consult an occupational therapist, who can advise you about options.

Hand Functions

Levers can be used to open or move a variety of objects such as lids on bottles and jars, door handles, or taps. It is easier to exert force, such as that involved in opening a door, if you use a lever. The pictures that follow show the difference in force needed to open a door with a round handle as compared to using a door handle that is a lever.

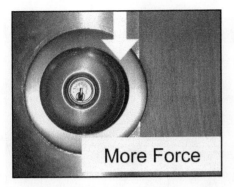

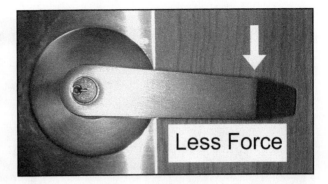

More Force

Less Force

TIP: *A small doorknob requires more force to open the door and uses smaller hand muscles; the longer lever handle requires less force and uses the larger forearm muscles.*

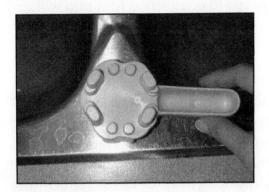

TIP: *Larger objects are easier to grasp and can cause less pain in the hands and fingers.*

A larger handgrip spreads the gripping force over many joints and reduces stress on any one area. It is also easier to hold and to use bigger objects, such as forks or spoons, that have sizable handles. Utensils and other household objects with larger handles are widely available. Adding foam padding to handles is a quick way to increase their size and improve the grip.

The large muscle groups in our legs, arms, and trunks are stronger than those in our fingers, feet, and ankles. Using these larger muscles helps produce more force with less effort and allows you to complete the task more efficiently. For example, it is easier to use your whole hand to grasp an object instead of trying to pinch it between your fingers and thumb.

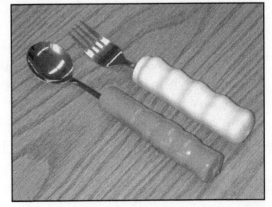

Chapter Seven | *Living in More Comfort: Maximizing Function and Energy*

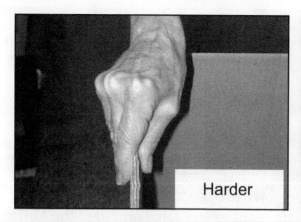
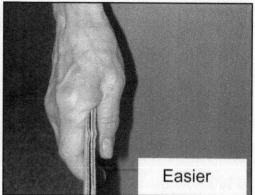

Harder

Easier

TIP: *Gripping as noted in the photo on the right uses larger muscles and decreases the amount of muscle force required to complete a task and will therefore assist in reducing pain.*

Cleaning the House

For most people, house cleaning is not a popular activity. Because of this, it is important that you do not try to do everything at once. Spring cleaning cannot be finished in a single day. Break up cleaning tasks and think about better ways to position yourself as you carry out the various activities. Simple cleaning products and devices reduce the amount of pressure needed in your hands for gripping and cut down on the reach required for activities such as vacuuming. It is common for people to complain of increased back or joint pain following vacuuming because the body is pushing and pulling with the back bent forward and the arms reaching. Vary these types of activities to give your body a rest from awkward or tiring positions. Also, think about the time of day that you do these chores. Avoid cleaning when you are fatigued or when you have more stiffness or pain than usual.

Assistive devices should be used to avoid excessive bending and stretching while cleaning. These tools allow you to stand straight while reaching for an object from the top shelf or picking up something from the floor. They help reduce the risk of back pain and injury when bending or stretching.

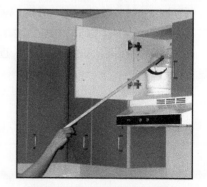

If you have hip or knee pain, using a long-handled mop is usually more comfortable than getting down on all fours and cleaning by hand. Remember, keep a neutral posture just as you do when vacuuming. Long handles can also be installed on window washers, dustpans, dusters, and other household tools.

Shopping

Here are some things to consider that can make shopping more comfortable. Before you leave for the store, put on a good pair of shoes that provide adequate support for your feet and have slip resistant tread. As you shop, take breaks, because walking on hard surfaces can be tiring. Whenever possible, use shopping carts with wheels to eliminate the strain of carrying items. Make sure the handle of the cart is at the right height so that you are not bending over. If no carts are available, try to carry only small, light packages. Also, look for shopping bags with wide hand grips; you may wish to purchase reusable cloth bags with wide hand grips that you can take with you on shopping trips. Finally, remember to get yourself and your bags in and out of the car safely, and be sure to lift groceries with as little strain as possible!

Leisure Time in Your Home

Think about the arrangement of your living room or the areas where you like to rest and relax. The height of chairs and couches should allow you to get up and down easily without excessive leg or arm work. Avoid low furniture, and consider using chairs that have arms, especially if your leg muscles are not strong or you have balance problems. Your arms and upper body are important for helping you move and balance your body as you get up and down. Having high, firm cushions on furniture makes it easier to move from sitting to standing. Avoid sitting in one position for long periods of time.

Recreational Activities

As noted in the chapter on exercise and physical activity (Chapter 6), there is solid evidence that individuals who are active have less pain and more energy. Follow the same principles outlined in that chapter when choosing or participating in a recreational activity.

Additional Guidelines to Improve Function while Reducing Pain

The suggestions above are designed to help you think more carefully about how you perform daily activities in your home and everyday life. Hopefully, some of these suggestions of adapting activities can improve your daily functioning while lessening your pain. In addition, you might find the following general guidelines to be helpful in managing your pain, regardless of your activities.

Lifting

Gardening, as well as other activities in the home, requires a fair amount of lifting. Lifting improperly can lead to back injuries that result in a good deal of pain. There are a few important things to remember when lifting objects around your home:

- Make sure that the object is light enough to lift safely.
- Get as close to the object as possible.
- Be sure to get a good grip.
- Keep a stable base of support with your feet flat on the ground and a good width apart.
- Bend at the knees, not at the trunk, and keep your back straight as you bend.
- Avoid twisting your trunk — turn by moving your feet.

If you have leg problems you should avoid lifting, as you will use other muscles excessively. These muscles are not effective for lifting, and using them this way can lead to further stress and pain.

Attempt to avoid lifting items over shoulder height as this puts excessive stress on the shoulder region, and also the neck and low back must often go into extreme positions, leading to risk of injury.

The Importance of Neutral Posture

Posture is a part of every activity (e.g., mowing the lawn), not just tasks that involve sitting or standing. In general, the body works most effectively and efficiently in a neutral position. Neutral body posture requires the least amount of muscle support, which produces minimal load on those muscles as well as the joints. The spine is not a straight rod; rather, it has four curves. Two of the curves in the neck and lower back curve in, while those in the mid-back and tail-bone curve out. These curves are necessary for proper functioning of the spine and should remain as close to normal as possible when standing, sitting, lifting, or bending. If these curves become too large or too small (i.e. flat), the spine may be put under too much stress, and pain or injury can result.

A neutral posture is achieved when (looking from the side) your ear, shoulder and hip are stacked one on top of the other, or a line drawn through these three points is straight. The four curves are what allow us to stand upright as shown here.

TIP: *Maintaining a neutral posture of the spinal regions while completing daily activities will help decrease the strain on your back and will therefore assist in reducing pain.*

Another way to assess your posture is to examine the position of your pelvis in a standing position. To locate the pelvis, put your hands on the right and left sides of your waist and then drop your hands down until you feel the top of the pelvic bone. The pelvis can tip either forward or back. If you think of it as a bucket of water, a neutral position is one in which the bucket is held upright so that no water spills out the front or back. Also, consider the position of the head on the spine. Don't poke out your chin when sitting or standing, as noted in the third picture on the next page.

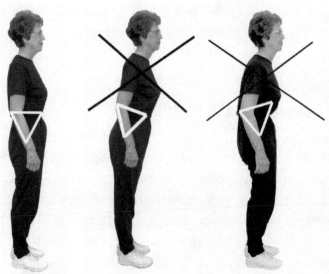

Try to maintain a neutral pelvic position—in other words, keep the water in the bucket—throughout your daily activities and whenever standing or sitting. If you use a walker or cane, make sure either one is fitted properly so that you can stand up straight and still have adequate support. It is essential to have walking devices properly fitted to your own body needs—have your physical therapist or other health professional appropriately assess your needs. People with certain physical problems or conditions, such as osteoporosis, may not be able to attain a neutral posture. These people should attempt to maintain a posture as close to the ideal as possible without feeling strain or discomfort.

Keep Objects Close

When you hold an object, keep it close to your body. The muscle force and joint forces are much less, which can assist in reducing pain.

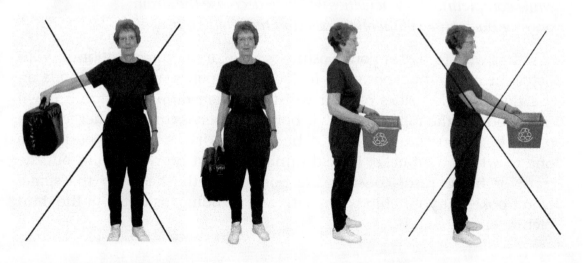

Change Position Frequently

Earlier in this chapter, we discussed ideal posture. Although this is the preferred position for your body, it is still not a good idea to stay in a stationary position for a long period of time. The body was made to move. Try to change your position frequently. For example, move from standing to sitting (or vice versa). If you are standing at the sink washing dishes for an extended period of time, try to take short breaks from this activity and do something else, then return to complete a bit more of the job after your break. When sitting, adjust your position often.

TIP: *Moving the joints frequently keeps them lubricated, prevents cramping of muscles and shortening of the surrounding tissues, and can decrease pain.*

If you purchase a new sofa or chair, think about the height of the seat. If the seat is too low or too soft you may be able to add a cushion or block under the cushion. Make sure this piece of furniture sits solidly on the floor. Higher seat cushions decrease the forces required from the large leg muscles when you sit or stand. Read the descriptions below for the easiest way to stand and sit using these larger muscles.

Standing Up. To stand, position yourself forward in your chair by shuffling to the edge of your seat. If you do not have good leg strength, use a chair with arms and put your hands firmly on the arms of the chair in order to use the arm muscles to assist you. The chair arms are helpful not only in providing force to lift and lower the body but also in helping to balance the body and prevent falls. Lean your body forward and keep your back in a neutral posture. Breathe in and out as you push yourself up, using your legs (see next page).

Sitting Down. Move to the front of your chair and turn slowly to face backwards to the chair, ideally with the back of your legs either touching or just a few inches from the seat. Place your feet about hip width apart and slowly bend at the hip and knees to lower your buttocks to the chair. Keep your back straight, allowing the hips, knees, and ankles to do the bending. Reach behind you so that the hands firmly contact the arms of your chair for support (if needed) as you lower yourself down using the muscles of your arms and legs (see next page).

115

Standing Up

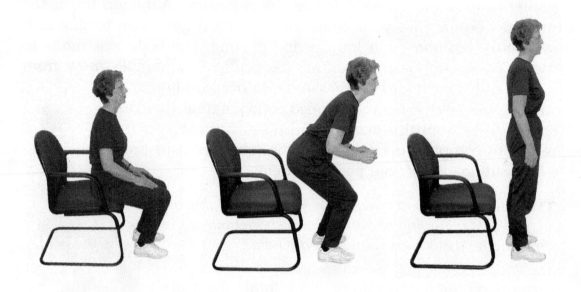

Sitting Down

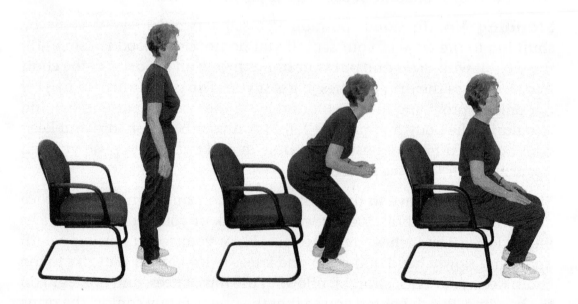

Chapter Seven | *Living in More Comfort: Maximizing Function and Energy*

Setting Up Your Work Spaces

If you use a computer or spend significant time at a desk, consider reading about efficient computer and office arrangement. The following are some general recommendations.

Purchase a comfortable computer chair that has adjustments for chair height and arm rests. The chair should be stable and allow you to position your feet flat on the floor. The knee position should be close to a 90-degree bend, which will help with good foot position and allow the body weight to be supported effectively through the legs. Use the up and down lever on the chair to find the right chair height for you. The setup of the computer and computer desk should be considered together so that the keyboard is positioned effectively to ensure that your wrists are in a relatively neutral position when typing. Also, it is essential that the height and the tilt of the computer monitor encourage a neck position that is not bent forward or backwards.

A well-lit room and an organized office will greatly assist with reducing soreness in the neck, low back, forearms, wrists, and fingers that could result from prolonged periods of using a computer in less than ideal positions. Take frequent breaks from your computer because not only do your eyes become fatigued, but your body needs to move to avoid

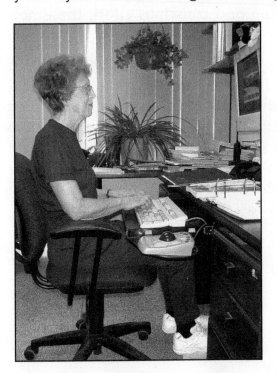

stiffness. Looking away from the computer screen for a few seconds is a good strategy, and so is getting up and walking around to give your back and your arms a break. A little easy stretching as described in Chapter 6 can be easily incorporated into the breaks.

117

Walking Devices and Wheelchairs

As we pointed out earlier, canes and walkers should be fitted properly. You should have appropriate instruction on how to use all walking devices. As simple as this may seem, using the walking device appropriately can make a significant difference in your comfort level and can also help minimize your pain. If you use a wheelchair, make sure that it fits the size of your body and is well maintained so that it is safe and efficient. If you need information about wheelchairs, your health professionals can refer you to the appropriate group that fits and services them.

Summary

As you read through the chapter, did you recognize any problems in the way you perform everyday activities (e.g., lifting or sitting at your computer) that might contribute to your chronic pain? If so, try to modify those activities and note the difference in your pain and energy levels. Keep in mind that this might require some conscious thought at first. For example, even though you now have a better idea about how to lift objects safely, you might occasionally forget and lift things the way you used to. With time and conscious effort, these new behaviors will become habits.

Similarly, were you able to spot any ways in which you might adjust your surroundings to ease your pain? In some cases, even simple changes (e.g., rearranging your kitchen so that heavier objects are not stored in bottom drawers or on the top shelves of cupboards) can make a big difference. Take the time to make these changes, and you'll be better off in the long run. Anything you can do to make your life easier and lower your chronic pain will be well worth the effort!

RONALD R. MARTIN, PHD, RD PSYCH.
SANDRA M. LEFORT, RN, PHD
STEPHANIE COOK, MSC, RD
SHANNON FUCHS-LACELLE, PHD

CHAPTER EIGHT

Sleep Hygiene and Nutrition

Sadie

Sadie, a 68-year-old woman, has experienced chronic pain in her right knee for the past year. Lately, she has been having trouble sleeping. Regardless of how tired she is, she goes to bed promptly at 9:30 every night but routinely lies awake for hours staring at the alarm clock. She often watches TV in her bedroom or turns on the VCR for the latest installment of an Agatha Christie series she has on tape. Before watching the tape, she fixes herself a sandwich and a drink. When she finally dozes off, the pain in her knee wakes her intermittently. She figures there is nothing she can do to make herself more comfortable. In the morning, she is so tired from her poor night's sleep that she ignores the alarm at 8:00 and sleeps in for an extra few hours. When she finally gets out of bed, she feels so tired she skips breakfast and instead drinks a pot of coffee. By lunchtime, she is famished and eats a large meal.

After reading about Sadie, you might ask yourself, *"What do sleep and nutrition have to do with chronic pain?"* Although it may not seem obvious now, sleep habits and diet are sometimes closely connected to many chronic pain problems. This chapter will help clarify these relationships. In your own experience, has pain ever interfered with your ability to get a good night's sleep? If so, you probably felt fatigued the next day. If this situation continues for more than a few days, you may find yourself feeling constantly exhausted, which makes coping with chronic pain even more difficult. If you experience either regular or occasional problems getting enough rest, this chapter will give you some helpful tips on how to improve the quality of your sleep.

Your diet may also be related to your pain. This chapter discusses certain types of foods that have been associated with both lower energy levels and increased chronic pain. As you learn about these types of foods, you will be encouraged to begin keeping track of how you feel after eating them. This will allow you to carefully examine the relationship between what you eat and how you feel!

Sleep and Chronic Pain

This section of the chapter addresses sleep problems. Difficulty getting proper rest may be common among older adults who experience chronic pain. The discussion that follows is intended to help you become more familiar with common sleep problems among older adults, gain a better understanding of sleep and its relationship to chronic pain, and learn how to use techniques that will help you sleep better.

Sleep Problems Can Increase with Age

Research indicates that problems with sleep get worse with age. From your own experience (and also considering other seniors you know), would you agree with the following?

- Many older adults (approximately 40%) report sleep difficulties.

- Older adults take longer to fall asleep.

- Seniors use medications (sleeping pills) to help them fall asleep more frequently than younger adults.

- Older adults wake up during the night more often than younger adults.

- Older adults spend more time in bed than younger adults but spend less time asleep than younger adults.

- Older women commonly have more trouble with their sleep than older men.

- Certain sleep disorders related to breathing or movement patterns become more common with age.

- Older adults spend less time in the "REM" stage of sleep (in which dreaming occurs) and in slow-wave (deeper) sleep, which means that they may wake up not feeling refreshed.

After reading the list of sleep problems experienced by seniors, you may wonder why such conditions occur more frequently among older than younger adults. The answer to this question is very complex and beyond the scope of this book. However, we can say that changes in sleep among older adults appear to be associated with multiple factors such as:

- Normal changes that occur with aging.

- Certain medical and psychological conditions (e.g., illnesses, depression).

- Life stressors (e.g., retirement, the death of a spouse).

- Bad sleep habits (e.g., too much caffeine before bedtime).

- Certain medications (sleeping pills).

- Pain that can interfere with the ability to fall asleep or stay asleep.

When faced with sleep problems, many older adults turn to sleeping pills for relief. Although sleeping pills are likely to work well initially, in some individuals they can interfere with sleep after prolonged use. Chronic (i.e., long-term) users of sleeping pills may find that, after a while, they need the drug just to get to sleep (this is known as "dependence"). Long-term users of sleeping pills may also find that they require more of the drug to achieve the same effect (this is known as "tolerance"). In some individuals, chronic use of sleeping pills may result in "withdrawal effects" (i.e., once you stop taking the sleeping pills, you may have trouble getting to sleep).

Ongoing, chronic use of sleeping pills can also have a negative impact on sleep quality. Before you begin taking sleeping pills, you should talk with your physician about the risks and benefits and the proper way to take the medication.

121

Chronic Pain and Sleep Problems

As we mentioned above, when you experience chronic pain, your sleep may be affected. Getting to sleep might be difficult because pain sometimes interferes with your ability to get comfortable. Also, once you have fallen asleep, your pain might wake you up. Getting back to sleep might be difficult if the pain is foremost in your mind. If you start to focus on your discomfort, you might begin to worry about losing sleep, especially if you have a busy schedule the following day. This increase in anxiety and worry sometimes makes it even more difficult to fall asleep. Anxiety and depression associated with chronic pain can also make it harder to fall asleep. Some people say that they experience "racing thoughts" that are not easily put to rest and can interfere with falling asleep.

Poor sleep may result in a number of undesirable consequences. These include stiff muscles, sleepiness, fatigue, memory and concentration problems, irritability, and sadness. These undesirable consequences of poor sleep leave older adults less able to cope with chronic pain. As a result, their sleep continues to be negatively affected by the pain, and a vicious circle begins to emerge.

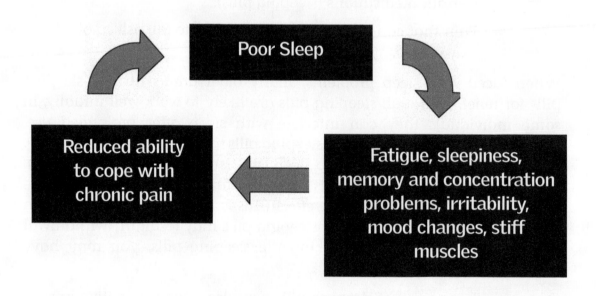

Sleep Hygiene: Cleaning Up Your Sleep Habits

Psychologists such as Patricia Lacks have outlined a variety of strategies to help improve sleep. This section describes a number of general guidelines and techniques that will help you to improve what is called *sleep hygiene.* Try following these guidelines and techniques to see if they make a difference for you. If you are able to make these changes part of your sleep routine, you will probably feel more refreshed and better able to manage your pain. To start off, let's go over the basics. The following considerations form the foundation of a good night's sleep.

When should you *head to bed?* The best time to go to bed at night is when you are sleepy. This may sound like common sense, but occasionally you might go to bed when you are still wide awake just because it's bedtime. In those instances, you could lie in bed awake for hours *trying* to get to sleep. A better strategy is to look for signs that your body is ready for sleep (such as frequent yawning and drooping eyelids).

Establish a bedtime routine. By establishing a routine before you go to bed, your body will learn to recognize a pattern of activities that precede sleep. As you carry out your bedtime routine, your body will recognize the sequence of activities as a cue that sleep is drawing near. This will help you to *wind down* automatically right before bedtime. Your bedtime routine might consist of a variety of activities, such as listening to relaxing music, brushing your teeth, and changing into your bed clothes.

Choose a regular wake-up time. It is understandable that your chronic pain might keep you awake and disrupt your sleep from time to time. Although it may be tempting to sleep later in the morning, it is vital that you maintain a consistent wake-up time. Changing your wake-up time (e.g., by sleeping in) disturbs your body's natural sleep rhythms and might make it more difficult for you to sleep at night.

Avoid taking naps. After a bad night's sleep, you might be tempted to take a nap the following day. Although a nap might feel great, your sleep will probably suffer the next night. It is like snacking before a meal: The more you snack, the less hungry you will be. The same principle applies to your sleep: The more you nap, the less sleepy you will be. The end result is that your sleep will continue to be disrupted. Thus, avoid naps during the day, and sleep will come more easily at night.

PRECAUTION: *Avoid driving when feeling sleepy. Sleepiness increases the risk of accidents.*

DO's and DON'Ts in the Bedroom

DO: Reserve the bedroom for sleeping and intimacy. The reason is that your brain makes associations between places and things. Ideally, the bedroom should be associated only with sleep and intimacy.

DON'T: Do not engage in stimulating activities (besides intimacy) in the bedroom, such as reading interesting stories, watching TV, or listening to the radio. These activities tend to hold our attention and activate us. Over time, your brain will associate the bedroom with being awake and engaged in these activities, which will make it difficult to get to sleep.

DO: If you don't fall asleep within 15 to 20 minutes, leave your bedroom and go to a different part of your home. This is important because you want your brain to associate the bedroom only with sleep and intimacy. Once in another area, do a relaxing activity (e.g., listening to soft music). Look for signs that your body is ready for sleep (e.g., frequent yawns, heavy eyelids), then go back to bed. If you are not asleep within 15 to 20 minutes, get up, leave the bedroom again, and repeat the process.

DON'T: *Trying* to fall asleep, or worrying about being awake, is not productive. Getting up is the most helpful thing you can do. The first week or two may be difficult for you. You may be getting up several times each night. As a result, you might not get much sleep initially. However, over time you should find that it's easier to get to sleep and stay asleep. To record your progress, fill out the sleep diary at the end of this chapter.

In addition to these *Do's and Don'ts,* another helpful suggestion is to examine your bedroom environment for conditions that will enhance or interfere with your ability to get quality sleep. Check the following in your bedroom.

Light sources. Try to eliminate sources of light in the bedroom by closing doors and adding drapes to windows. *Note:* Some digital alarm clocks have displays that may be too bright, and people suffering from insomnia tend to "watch the clock." Reduce the intensity of the display or turn it away from you.

Noise. Make sure there are no sources of noise in the bedroom. Problem solve in order to reduce any noises that are specific to your household (e.g., fix or replace household fixtures or appliances that make intermittent noise when you are trying to sleep). Also, there are many different kinds of earplugs that you might try. Find a comfortable pair that reduces noise and improves your sleep.

Temperature. Choose a room temperature that makes it easier for you to sleep. Increase or decrease the number of blankets as necessary until you find your optimum comfort level.

Mattress. Make sure that your mattress is the best quality you can afford. There are no absolute guidelines about the firmness—some people prefer a firm bed, while others prefer a softer place to sleep. In choosing or altering the firmness of your mattress, your doctor, chiropractor, or physical therapist may be able to give you advice that is specific to your needs.

Pillows. You may find it helpful to use small pillows to ease stress on certain parts of your body. If you have back pain, lying on your side with a small pillow between your knees may help to take the stress off your low back and hips. Small pillows may also provide additional comfort and support to parts of your body that give you pain.

In addition to the recommendations above, there are certain things you should try to avoid right before going to bed since they might interfere with sleep.

Avoid eating or drinking too much. In general, you should avoid eating large meals or drinking a lot of fluids immediately before bed. Indigestion, heartburn, and frequent trips to the bathroom will stand in the way of your getting an uninterrupted night's sleep.

Avoid stimulants. Two commonly used stimulants have been shown to affect sleep negatively: caffeine and nicotine.

Caffeine is the stimulant most people associate with coffee, but it is also found in tea, chocolate, and many soft drinks. Check the ingredient labels of foods and drinks you consume witin several hours of going to bed. Where possible, substitute caffeine-free foods and beverages. It's a small price to pay for a better night's sleep!

Nicotine is a stimulant found in tobacco products (e.g., cigarettes, pipe tobacco) and nicotine gums. Ingesting nicotine within several hours of your bedtime may disrupt your sleep.

Avoid alcoholic beverages. Some people use alcohol to relax and help them fall asleep. While alcohol may accomplish these goals in the short run, it may have a negative impact on the quality of your sleep by causing frequent awakenings if consumed within several hours of your bedtime.

Avoid exercising in the evening. Exercise before bed may have an energizing effect that interferes with your sleep. Try exercising earlier in the day in order to obtain the physical and mental benefits while preserving your sleep.

In addition to the recommendations and techniques above, there are other things that you might consider to improve your sleep. Try the following and note the results!

Relaxation techniques. A variety of relaxation techniques are covered in Chapter 3 that you might find helpful, such as diaphragmatic breathing or imagery exercises.

Soothe yourself. People with chronic pain often report that warm baths or compresses help to ease their pain. Other ways of soothing yourself include having a hot drink (noncaffeinated), looking at pleasant images, or listening to relaxing music. Individuals vary in terms of what they find relaxing. Take a moment to consider what things you find calming.

Exercise. Contrary to what you might think, exercise can benefit people who experience chronic pain (e.g., by improving cardiovascular fitness, strength, flexibility, and endurance). Exercise can also have beneficial effects on your sleep if you exercise in the morning or afternoon. However, vigorous physical activity in the evening may interfere with your sleep.

Consult your doctor to work out an exercise plan that is safe and effective for you (for more information, see Chapter 6). It is generally advised to refrain from strenuous physical exertion within several hours of bedtime since this will probably *activate* your body and keep you awake.

After reviewing the information in this chapter, Sadie decided to make several changes to her sleep habits. She changed her bedtime from 9:30 to 11:00 p.m. Before bed, she now routinely takes a warm bath. Alternatively, she turns on some light music for about 15 minutes. She removed the TV and VCR from her bedroom. She bought herself a new pillow, something she figured she deserved since it had been at least 15 years since she'd had a new one. After making these changes, Sadie now consistently gets out of bed at 7:00 a.m.

Nutrition and Chronic Pain

This section addresses the relation between nutrition and chronic pain. Although it may seem strange at first, the foods you eat can have an impact on the pain you experience. This section reviews the importance of a good diet and provides basic information about nutrition as well as the relationship between nutrition and ongoing pain.

A healthy diet is important for several reasons. In general, eating a balanced diet enhances general health and fitness. It helps us to maintain our proper weight while looking and feeling our best. A sound diet not only enables us to perform at optimal levels but also reduces fatigue. It even helps diminish problems like constipation (which can aggravate back pain), medication side effects (especially stomach and intestinal problems), and certain diseases (e.g., heart disease, high blood pressure, diabetes, some kinds of cancers, and osteoporosis). Clearly, the quality of your diet can have a big impact on your health and your quality of life!

Malnutrition

In extreme cases, the consequences of a poor diet may include malnutrition. Although malnutrition is rare in community-dwelling seniors, the rates increase as health and functional abilities decrease. According to a Health Canada document entitled *Dare to Age Well! Healthy Aging: Nutrition and Healthy Aging,* malnutrition is associated with lower resistance to infection, decreased body strength, and poor quality of life. Further, low body weight (in proportion to one's height) and excessive weight loss may be associated with hip fractures. Injuries such as these may result in reduced independence, early admission to long-term care, and increased mortality rates.

Being Overweight

Being overweight can have a negative effect on health in general but can also aggravate several types of joint or muscle pain. Excess weight, for example, puts more stress on the knees. Overweight persons with joint problems will typically have more pain difficulties than those who are not overweight. The good news is that even losing a relatively small amount of excess weight can substantially reduce joint stress and joint-related problems. If you are overweight, do not hesitate to consult with a dietitian or other qualified professional for personalized advice. The dietitian may also encourage you to join a weight loss program in your community.

It is important to be aware that excess body weight can sometimes result from medical conditions (e.g., hormonal problems). If necessary, your doctor will be able to order tests to determine if hormonal or other medical factors are interfering with the maintenance of a healthy weight.

Keys to Healthy Weight Control

If you are overweight, here are a few tips to start you on the road to success with long-term weight control.

Set realistic goals. Aim for a gradual weight loss of no more than 1 to 2 pounds (0.5 to 1 kg) per week. To do this, gradually modify your eating habits and make practical changes that you can live with permanently.

Practice portion control. Moderation is the key to cutting down on your food intake, but be sure to continue eating a variety of foods each day. Remember that all foods can be enjoyed—even the higher-calorie ones, in moderation. The best way to practice portion control is to learn what serving sizes and portions actually look like (e.g., a serving of meat is 100 grams or about 3 ounces, which is the same size as a deck of cards).

Balance your food intake over the day. Develop an eating schedule. Try to have three meals a day and avoid skipping meals, which often leads to overeating later. To prevent swings in your blood sugar, which can lead to feelings of hunger and cravings for sweets, each meal should include a starch food (such as whole-wheat bread, whole-wheat pasta, or brown rice) along with a protein (such as lean meat, chicken, fish, or low-fat cheese).

Choose lower-fat foods. Everyone needs some fat in his or her diet, but most people eat too much. Using the lower-fat versions of foods such as dairy products, mayonnaise, and salad dressings can go a long way to reducing your fat intake. Some other useful strategies to help you decrease your fat intake include avoiding fried foods as well as snacks such as corn or potato chips and chocolate.

Gradually increase your activity level. Look for ways to increase your activity level that fit your daily routine.

General Nutritional Guidelines

The best way to make sure you are getting balanced nutrition is to eat a variety of nutrient-rich foods every day. It is important to stay within your daily calorie needs, which are determined by your age, body size, and activity level. Most people require fewer calories as they age. However, it is still important to ensure that you get all the nutrients you need. This presents an interesting challenge: How do you get adequate nutrients in a smaller number of calories? The best way is to practice the following recommendations for healthy eating.

Know the facts. Most packaged foods have a Nutrition Facts label. Healthy eating starts at the grocery store where you can use this label information to make better food choices. Be sure to check the serving size and make your calories count. This means looking at the calories on the label and comparing them to the nutrients (e.g., vitamins, calcium) you are getting. The best choices are foods that pack the most nutrients into the fewest calories.

Eat plenty of fruits and vegetables. Eating a variety of fruits and vegetables is the cornerstone of a healthy diet. Choose more dark green vegetables, such as broccoli, kale, and spinach, and more orange ones such as carrots, sweet potatoes, and squash. Both varieties are loaded with important nutrients.

Focus on whole-grain breads and cereals. At least half of the grains you eat should be "whole." This means choosing at least three servings of whole-grain cereals, breads, rice, and pasta every day. Read the ingredient list on the foods you select to be sure that they contain whole grains.

Reduce fat added to cooking and at the table. Try to limit the obvious fats, such as butter, margarine, oil, peanut butter, gravy, salad dressings, and mayonnaise to no more than six servings each day. Limit your choice of fats to those which contain vegetable oils (olive, canola, or peanut oil), and avoid foods that contain saturated fat, *trans* fat, or are "hydrogenated."

Select lean meats, poultry, fish and alternatives. Limit your intake of lean meat and poultry to no more than 100 to 200 grams per day (6 to 8 ounces). Meat alternatives, such as beans and lentils, are healthier options and should be included more often. Fish is also an important part of a healthy diet because it contains omega-3 fatty acids (i.e., fish oils) that help reduce the risk of heart disease. However, because of concerns with mercury exposure, avoid fish such as shark, swordfish, mackerel, and fresh or frozen tuna. Include up to two servings of fish such as wild salmon, pollock, sole, catfish, or shrimp each week.

Choose lower-fat dairy products. Dairy products are the best source of calcium, a nutrient important for healthy bones. Look for milk, yogurt, and cottage cheese that contain 2% milk fat or less, as well as low-fat cheeses with no more than 15% milk fat. Aim for three servings of low-fat dairy products every day.

Avoid high-fat desserts and snacks. The fat and calories we consume in the form of desserts and snacks can quickly add up. Try snacking on fruits or vegetables or look for healthier alternatives such as angel food cake, popcorn, sherbet, yogurt, and puddings. Avoid high-fat foods such as pastries, doughnuts, commercial muffins, cakes, cookies, chips, and chocolate.

Know the limits on salt and sugar. In addition to reading the Nutrition Facts label for information on the serving size, fat, and calories, be sure to choose foods and beverages with little salt and added sugar. A good guide for sodium is to aim for less than 2300 milligrams per day. Sugars contribute calories with very few nutrients. Look for foods in which sugar (including sucrose, glucose, evaporated cane juice, corn syrup, and high-fructose corn syrup) is not listed as one of the first few ingredients.

Other Foods and Beverages to Consider if You Have Chronic Pain

There is no specific diet for people with ongoing pain. Rather, the best course of action is to follow an overall plan for healthy eating that provides you with all the nutrients you need to meet your requirements and feel energetic. However, the foods you eat can have an impact on your mental and physical health. You may find that some foods and caffeinated beverages can affect your pain. These are described in more detail below. Before you read on, there are two key points that you should keep in mind. First, any changes you make to your diet should be gradual. Second, it is usually a good idea to make such changes one at a time. This helps you understand how each individual dietary change affects your pain and your overall health and well-being.

Caffeine. Caffeine, a mild stimulant, is present in many of our favorite foods and beverages such as coffee (the most popular beverage in the world), tea, chocolate, and many soft drinks. Many over-the-counter drugs, particularly painkillers, also contain caffeine. Popular as it is, caffeine can make people restless and anxious. It is also known to produce noticeable physical problems such as heart palpitations and stomach distress. These negative effects can worsen your chronic pain (e.g., by altering the quality of your sleep). If you are consuming too much caffeine and you would like to cut back, you should do so over a period of weeks. Eliminating caffeine too quickly might result in *withdrawal* symptoms such as headache, nausea, nervousness, reduced alertness, or mood changes. Try switching gradually to decaffeinated coffees and teas. Also, read medication labels carefully or check with your pharmacist to determine whether the medications you are taking contain caffeine.

Alcohol. Some people who experience chronic pain use alcohol to numb their discomfort. While alcohol may reduce pain temporarily, turning to alcohol for relief is a bad idea for several reasons. First, alcohol relaxes your muscles, but it does not act as a painkiller. Second, it dilates your blood vessels, which can bring on migraines or headaches. Alcohol is also an addictive (habit-forming) drug. Since it is a depressant, it may worsen pain and may even cause depression once its effects have worn off. Alcohol in moderation (i.e., one drink per day) is sometimes recommended; however, you may find that even moderate consumption can lead to a worsening of your pain and your mood. If you have been drinking large amounts of alcohol for an extended period of time, talk with your doctor about reducing or eliminating your consumption.

MSG (monosodium glutamate). MSG is a flavor enhancer often added to foods such as sauces, soups, prepared meals, and ethnic foods. Considerable debate has taken place about whether MSG is responsible for such symptoms as headaches, migraines, and tightness in the chest. This group of symptoms is often referred to as *Chinese Restaurant Syndrome* because MSG is so commonly used in Asian cuisine. In actual fact, research has not found a definitive link between MSG and any of these health effects. However, if you want to moderate your MSG intake, or if you seem sensitive to it, be sure to read the Nutrition Facts labels to determine if foods contain MSG. Sometimes this is tricky because terms such as *natural flavor, flavor,* or *hydrolyzed vegetable protein* may mean that MSG is present. When ordering foods from restaurants, ask if the meal contains MSG. If it does, find out if the chef can prepare your meal without this additive.

Aspartame. One of the most often used food additives, aspartame (marketed under the brand name NutraSweet) is found in a variety of products including soft drinks, yogurt, puddings, frozen desserts, and candy. Since its discovery in 1965, aspartame has been thoroughly investigated, and an overwhelming amount of research has concluded that it is safe. However, many people have reported that aspartame triggers headaches and migraines. If you think you may be sensitive to aspartame, keep a food diary to determine if there is a link between your pain and such additives. Fortunately, foods containing aspartame are easy to spot since manufacturers must identify it on the label or ingredient list.

Chocolate, red wine, aged cheese, and preservatives. It is possible that specific components of foods, both those that occur naturally or those that have been added, may cause migraine headaches in some people. Tyrosine (found in aged cheese and chocolate), histamine (found in red wine), and benzoic acid (a preservative) may be the components responsible.

The best way to determine if a food component is triggering your pain is to keep a diary of what you eat (see the *Food Challenge* diary at the end of this chapter). However, it can sometimes be difficult to determine which ingredients or components of foods you may be sensitive to. If you think you may have a reaction to something in your diet, a registered dietitian can assist you in sorting this out. To help you review this information, we have included a nutrition review sheet on page 138.

Sadie reviewed the above information and generally found that she was making sound nutritional decisions. She admitted, however, that she ate at irregular periods throughout the day and often snacked late at night. At first, she tried being consistent by having three regular mealtimes each day along with two light snacks, one in the mid-afternoon and one at 8:00 p.m. Then she stopped eating past 8:00 p.m., especially right before bed. After making this change for several weeks, Sadie noticed that her energy level was more stable throughout the day. She then decided to reduce her coffee consumption to two cups of coffee or tea in the morning. Although she found this change a bit more difficult to make, within a week she was sleeping better and was not feeling the need to drink several cups of coffee in the morning.

Summary

Now that you've finished this chapter, we hope you will make use of the suggestions you've read here. After all, getting a good night's sleep on a regular basis is one of the foundations of effective pain management. Also, take the time to use the exercises at the end of the chapter to better understand the relationships between pain and your sleeping and eating habits. Monitor how you feel after eating certain foods or drinking beverages that contain caffeine. This will help you identify which specific foods negatively affect your energy levels, your chronic pain, and other aspects of your physical and mental health. Also, try keeping track of these foods and your pain levels with the help of the *Food Challenge* monitoring form on page 139. At the very least, we hope that this chapter will encourage you to follow a healthier diet!

Sleep Habits

Use the following questions to help you improve your sleep habits.

1. What time does your body begin to show signs of being ready for sleep (e.g., yawning, drooping eyelids)?

    _____

2. What activities could be part of your bedtime routine (e.g., brushing teeth, changing into bed clothes, doing a relaxation strategy)?

    _____

3. What time would be a regular wake-up time for you?

    _____

4. Which of the following do you need to stop doing to improve your sleep?

    ____ Taking naps

    ____ Lying in bed for more than 15 minutes when not able to sleep

    ____ Drinking too much liquid before bed

    ____ Having too much caffeine during the day

    ____ Watching television in bed

    ____ Lying in bed worrying

    ____ Drinking too much coffee, tea, or cola during the day

    ____ Drinking alcohol before bed

    ____ Reading in bed

    ____ Eating before going to bed

    ____ Smoking too much during the day

    ____ Exercising in the evening

5. Which of the following do you need to do to improve your sleep environment?

    ____ Reduce sources of light   ____ Adjust room temperature   ____ Change the mattress

    ____ Decrease noise level   ____ Change the number of blankets   ____ Use different pillows

6. Could you use the following strategies to help you sleep?

    ____ Relax your muscles   ____ Focus on relaxing images   ____ Practice deep breathing

    ____ Exercise during the morning or afternoon   ____ Listen to relaxing music   ____ Take a warm bath before bed

Sleep Diary

Use this diary to monitor your progress as you are working toward improving the quality of your sleep.

Date day/month/year	What time did you go to bed?	Did you go to bed when you were tired?	If you did not get to sleep in 15 minutes or less, did you get up and leave the bedroom?	How many times did you get up and leave the bedroom?	What did you do when you left the bedroom?	What time did you wake up the next morning?

Nutrition Review

Mark True or False beside each statement below. For the items you answer false, consider making one change each week. For instance, this week you might focus on limiting your salt intake. Next week, you could try eating more fruits and vegetables.

_____ I read the Nutrition Facts label when grocery shopping to help me select healthier foods.

_____ I eat a variety of fruits and vegetables each day.

_____ I have three servings of low-fat dairy products each day.

_____ I limit my intake of meat and poultry to two servings each day.

_____ I choose at least one vegetable that is dark green or orange each day.

_____ I focus on whole grains rather than processed foods.

_____ I use less salt.

_____ I limit the alcohol I drink.

_____ I cut back on caffeine.

_____ I don't add as much sugar to my food.

_____ I choose lower-fat dairy products.

_____ I eat meat alternatives such as fish, beans, and lentils more often.

_____ I cut down on my use of butter, margarine, and dressing.

_____ I bake or broil my foods more often.

_____ I use light broths and herbs to season my food.

_____ I avoid deep-fried foods.

_____ I avoid snacks like chips and chocolate bars.

_____ I eat three meals a day.

_____ I avoid eating food with MSG.

_____ I stay away from foods with aspartame.

_____ I avoid preservatives.

Food Challenge

Remember, your chronic pain may worsen because of a sensitivity to some of the things you eat or because of factors such as hormonal changes. Other stressors (e.g., conflict with others, feeling depressed) may also intensify pain. The use of the monitoring form below may help you identify and eliminate the foods that lead to, or worsen, your pain.

Use this pain rating scale for the Food Challenge form:

0 = no pain	1 = mild	2 = discomforting
3 = distressing	4 = horrible	5 = excruciating

Food or drink	Date and time of pain	Location or type of pain	Pain rating (0 to 5)		
			Before eating	After eating	Several hours later
Example: coffee	*15/12/07 3:00 p.m.*	*migraine*	*0*	*0*	*4*

CHAPTER NINE

Effective Communication with Your Doctor

Have you ever gone to the doctor with a mental list of problems, only to forget several important details once the appointment has ended? Have you ever had difficulty recalling important information (e.g., the onset, duration, or severity of a medical problem) when the doctor asks you for specific details?

These scenarios are common. In a perfect world, you would have plenty of time at each doctor's appointment, but experience tells us that most visits are extremely brief! So, you must do your best to make the most of the time you have with your physician. This requires some preparation. One of the most important things you can do to help manage your pain is to become an *active* partner on your health care team. While it is likely that there are many health care providers involved with your treatment, your relationship with your doctor is an important one. This chapter will provide you with specific suggestions on what you can do to plan for your doctor's visits so that you make good use of your limited time!

The Doctor-Patient Relationship

Researchers have known for a long time that a good doctor–patient relationship is essential to receiving high-quality health care. However, the need for a good doctor–patient relationship is especially important

141

when it involves chronic pain, since an understanding of the causes for pain and its treatment are not always widely agreed upon.

A good doctor–patient relationship can be vital to your diagnosis and treatment. What doctors know about their patients and the pain they experience is generally based on the doctor's interpretation of patients' words, appearance, and behaviors. Research has shown that much of a pain diagnosis is based on what the patient tells his or her doctor, while very little is based on the physical exam. So, be sure to tell your doctor about your pain! Some patients are comfortable describing their pain to their doctor. However, many people downplay their pain to put on a brave front, especially if the pain is chronic or getting worse.

As humans, we want to be liked. This need is no different when it comes to our relationship with our doctor. However, by minimizing your pain, you limit your doctor's ability to diagnose and treat it accurately. Dealing with pain involves trust. Knowing that you can talk honestly with your doctor about your concerns will make you feel more comfortable. For example, some patients feel a sense of embarrassment or failure if their pain is not responding to the prescribed treatment. When this happens, they are reluctant to tell the doctor. Having a good doctor–patient relationship will allow you to communicate openly about your symptoms and treatment progress. This type of communication will help you feel more satisfied afterward and can help you achieve better results.

Because the time you have with your doctor is short, it may be hard to share all of the information you would like. You may not be able to ask all the questions you have. Patients who take time to plan their visits generally have a better relationship with their doctor.

The advice that follows can help you get more out of your doctor's visit and will allow you to participate in your health care as a partner.

Preparing for Your Appointment

Asking questions and sharing information about your condition and treatment are two important ways to develop a good doctor–patient relationship. While this may sound simple, it can be difficult for patients. For example, some people believe that their doctor should be in charge, and they don't like to ask questions. Others think that when they try to share information about their pain with their doctor, they will be accused of being hypochondriacs or drug seekers. Still others may feel that their questions are too silly or embarrassing to ask. However, it is important to remember that most doctors want you to ask questions and share information about yourself. The doctor has probably heard similar questions to the ones you will ask, so you are not likely to surprise him or her.

One way to make sure you get the answers to your questions is to make a list of things you would like to talk about with your doctor. This list may include questions about your pain symptoms, medications you are taking, or family history that may be important. Making a list will keep you from forgetting anything. Also, make sure you bring all the medications you are taking, including prescriptions and other medications or supplements (e.g., vitamins, glucosamine). Providing information about your pain and your response to treatment is also critical. For example, if you are experiencing a change in your pain, your doctor will want to know when the change began, where it occurred, and any changes in your life that may be affecting the change (e.g., lifestyle, stress level, new herbal therapies, and exercises).

Remembering this kind of information can be hard. Some people, however, find that keeping a daily diary (see Chapter 2) is a helpful way to remember important health-related matters. A daily diary can help you keep track of changes in your pain and is also a great place to write down questions you would like your doctor to answer. You could also make copies of the pain diary to take with you on your visit.

At the Visit

The visit with your doctor will most likely be short. When you arrive, tell your doctor what you would like to talk about. Find out what he or she wants to discuss. If you cannot cover everything that day, the two of you can decide together what is most important and what will have to be covered at another visit.

The doctor will have specific questions for you regarding your pain symptoms and response to treatment. Be certain to share all of the details. Even if something does not seem related to your symptoms, share as much information as you have.

Your doctor needs to know:

- *What you think is going on and why.*
- *Anything you have learned so far about the problem and its treatment.*
- *Whatever you have tried so far to get better.*
- *Your biggest concerns related to the problem.*
- *Whether your pain has gotten better or worse since treatment began.*

Taking notes during your appointment will help you remember what was said. Some people bring a family member or friend for emotional support, and this person can also write down any important information.

Most people don't understand all of the medical terms used by doctors. If you have trouble with any of the terms or instructions, ask your doctor to repeat them in a way you can understand. Some people find that learning some basic medical terminology helps them feel more comfortable when talking with their doctor. Ask if there are any pamphlets or information sheets that you can take home. Some pharmacies have audio- or video cassettes that you can borrow. The library and the Internet are also great resources for getting more information on your condition.

If the doctor is talking too fast, ask him or her to slow down. Repeat what you think you heard to check your understanding. Asking questions and repeating instructions are two important ways that tell your doctor that you understand what he or she has said. But if this still fails to make things clear, ask that all health-related instructions be written out for you.

After the Visit

After your visit, read the notes you took. A journal or diary is a good way to keep track of your doctor visits. Write down what you learned, for example, about your prescribed medications and other treatment options. If you have more questions, phone or visit your doctor again.

If you are told that you need certain tests, be sure you understand what will happen at the test and when it will occur. Know what this examination will involve, whether you will experience any pain or discomfort, how to prepare, and why the doctor is requesting the test. Let the doctor know you would like to be informed of the results even if they show that nothing is wrong. Ask when you can have the results, and follow up with your doctor if you have not heard anything by that time.

You might have a choice of treatments, so be sure to discuss the options with the doctor. If medications are prescribed, learn what they are, how they will help, and whether they have side effects.

Finally, make sure you know how to follow the recommended treatment plan and understand how it will help your condition.

Sample Questions

Below are some questions that you may want to ask your doctor. Before your next appointment, review these questions, or bring this sheet with you!

About your condition:

- *What has happened to me?*
- *Why did it happen?*
- *Did I do something to cause it?*
- *How long will I have this condition?*

About your treatment options:

- *What do I need to do now?*
- *What choices do I have in treating the condition?*
- *What are the good things about each choice?*
- *What are the bad things about each choice?*
- *Will they hurt? How much?*

About your medical tests:

- *What is the name of the test/procedure?*
- *What will it tell you?*
- *How long will it last? Will it hurt?*
- *Where and when will I have the test?*
- *What should I do to prepare?*

About your medical tests (continued)

- ◎ *Can I eat and drink before the test?*
- ◎ *Do I need to take any medicine beforehand?*
- ◎ *Is it all right to take my regular medications prior to the test?*
- ◎ *Will I need to have someone take me home afterwards?*
- ◎ *What will happen if I decide not to have it done?*
- ◎ *When can I call you for the results?*

About referrals:

- ◎ *Why do I need to see a specialist?*
- ◎ *What kind of specialist do I need?*
- ◎ *What will he or she do?*
- ◎ *Who will be in charge of my treatment?*
- ◎ *How will the specialist work with my doctor?*
- ◎ *Who will choose the specialist?*
- ◎ *What will happen if I don't see the specialist?*

About your medication:

- ◎ *What is the name of my medication?*
- ◎ *Why am I taking it? What is it for?*
- ◎ *Do you have any samples of the drug for me to try before I fill my prescription?*
- ◎ *Is there a generic brand?*
- ◎ *Is this prescription covered by my drug plan?*
- ◎ *How often should I take it?*
- ◎ *When should I take it? Before, after, or with meals? At bedtime? As needed?*
- ◎ *Are there any specific foods or beverages I should avoid?*
- ◎ *Are there any over-the-counter medications I should avoid taking at the same time?*
- ◎ *What side effects might I experience while taking this drug?*
- ◎ *How long should I take it?*
- ◎ *What are the expected results?*

Summary

How would you rate your satisfaction with your doctor's appointments? If there are things about these visits that you find unsatisfying, the contents of this chapter may help you to turn things around. The suggestions outlined above are offered to help you to get the basic information you need to make informed decisions and to receive the best care possible. You deserve nothing less! See the section below and on the next page for a review of the steps to take before, during, and after your medical appointment.

Guidelines for Your Medical Appointment

Before the Appointment:

- *Make a list of subjects you want to discuss with your doctor at your next appointment.*

- *From this list, choose the two or three things that are most important to you.*

- *Collect all your medications in a bag and bring them to the appointment.*

- *Consider bringing a family member or good friend.*

- *Review your pain diary (Chapter 2) and consider showing it to your doctor.*

At the Appointment:

- *Discuss with your doctor which questions the two of you can cover during the current visit.*

- *Share as many details as possible regarding your concerns.*

- *If you don't understand what your doctor is saying, ask him or her to repeat the information in a way you can understand.*

- *Ask whether your doctor would like to see a copy of your pain diary.*

- *Ask questions and take notes.*

- *Repeat back what you think your doctor said to make sure you understand.*

After the Appointment:

- ◎ *Review your notes.*

- ◎ *Be certain you understand your treatment. Ask more questions about any recommended tests, medications, or additional treatment options.*

- ◎ *Keep your doctor informed of any changes in your condition.*

- ◎ *Make an appointment to discuss any concerns that your doctor did not have time to cover during your appointment.*

ROMAYNE GALLAGHER, MD, CCFP
B. LYNN BEATTIE, MD, FRCP(C)
RONALD R. MARTIN, PHD, RD PSYCH.

CHAPTER TEN

The Role of Medications

Have you ever felt confused about all the medication options that are available for the treatment of pain? Have you had difficulty finding answers to questions you have about different drugs? Given that so many analgesics (painkillers) are currently available, this chapter will help you gain a better understanding of the many options and will explain the process that health professionals use to control your pain effectively.

This chapter will also discuss the following topics:

- *The role of medications*
- *General pain management rules*
- *Pain medications (i.e., analgesics)*
- *Classes of pain medication:*
  - *Non-opioids*
  - *Nonsteroidal anti-inflammatory drugs (NSAIDs)*
  - *Opioids*
- *Other medications for pain*
- *Anesthesia interventions*
- *Future directions in pain management*
- *Pain-related conditions that are common among seniors*

PRECAUTION: This information is for educational purposes only and is not a substitute for medical advice. Be sure to discuss with your physician any and all medications that you are currently taking or are thinking about taking. Please also see the disclaimer in the front pages of this book.

149

The Role of Medications

The goal of analgesics is to reduce pain to a level that allows you to function physically and emotionally and as independently as possible. The challenge in using medications is to strike a balance between the most effective relief of pain and the fewest side effects.

Since so many people turn to medications for help with pain relief, it is helpful to get a better understanding of some general pain management guidelines. The use of pain drugs, along with the reassessment of the pain and adjustment of the dosage, is a dynamic process that requires the input of patient, caregiver, and health care professional. The dosage must be changed according to the intensity of pain, duration of pain relief, type of pain, side effects of the drug, and the metabolism of the individual. Your health care professional will want you to note how much pain you are feeling, how much relief you get from your medication, and how long it lasts.

If you suffer from constant pain, you will most likely need regular medication. Medications are often prescribed on a regular basis in an effort to break the cycle of overwhelming pain and to keep ahead of severe pain. Pain can vary widely during the day, and there are times when your pain may increase beyond your comfort level. When this happens, you can take more of the medication. This is called *breakthrough* or *rescue* medication and serves to reduce the pain to a manageable level. Often, when pain gets *out of control,* it takes more medication and more time to get it back under control than if you had prevented the pain from building up in the first place.

Take your medications according to the dosing schedule (e.g., *take X number of pills every X hours*). If the schedule is properly managed, your next dose should occur before the pain-relieving effects of the last one wear off. It is important for your doctor to know if this is working because it helps determine the right schedule for you.

Medications must be taken as prescribed. Sometimes people do not take their pills when they should, either because they forget or because they find the directions confusing. If you have difficulties following instructions with regard to your medications, your health care professionals have ways of simplifying things for you. For example, *bubble packing* is a system where the pharmacist packages all the pills for a week in an easy-to-read card with plastic *bubbles* that contain the pills for each specific day and/or time.

Some people may not feel comfortable taking a certain medication. They may misunderstand what the medication is meant to do or have concerns about side effects. If you need to know more about the drugs you are taking, be sure to ask your health care professional. Some concerns arise from misleading information. For example, concerns over a high rate of addiction with morphine and other opioid pain relievers tend to be exaggerated.

People often take a great deal of over-the-counter medication when they feel pain. Large doses of these nonprescription medications, taken in addition to prescription medications, can result in overuse and potentially ineffective long-term pain management. If you are considering taking any over-the-counter pain relievers, speak with your physician first.

In addition to understanding the general pain management guidelines described in this section, you may find it helpful to learn more about formal strategies for choosing pain medications. The following section outlines a pain medication selection strategy that was developed by the World Health Organization.

Analgesics (Pain Medications): Rationale for Selection

The World Health Organization (WHO) developed the *analgesic ladder* in 1984 to define a rational approach to the use of pain medication and to improve pain management (see the next page for a graphical representation of this approach). The original use of the *stepwise* approach was for cancer pain, but the approach can now be used for any chronic pain condition. This stepped approach recommends giving medication according to the intensity of the pain and the effect of the medication. For example, someone may have pain in his or her knees from osteoarthritis. He or she may have tried the maximum dose of acetaminophen (paracetamol), but the pain may still be out of control. At this point, the doctor may advise a step up to a stronger drug such as acetaminophen with oxycodone.

The doctor may also suggest that an antidepressant drug be tried. An antidepressant is an example of an adjuvant pain medication — a drug that relieves pain as an extra effect in addition to the one it is primarily used for. Other adjuvant pain medications are anticonvulsants, anesthetics, antispasmodics, and other less common drugs.

If an adequate trial of these medications does not relieve the pain sufficiently, then a stronger opioid might be used with or without continuing the antidepressant. In addition, complementary approaches, such as those mentioned in other chapters of this book, should be pursued.

Rationale for Selection of Pain Medication
(Based on work by the World Health Organization)

Step 1. Non-opioid

Possible use of adjuvant

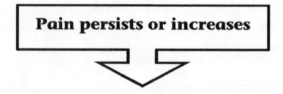

Pain persists or increases

Step 2. Opioid suitable for *mild to moderate* pain

Possible use of non-opioid

Possible use of adjuvant

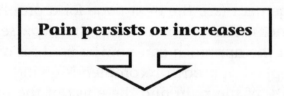

Pain persists or increases

Step 3. Opioid suitable for moderate to severe pain

Possible use of non-opioid

Possible use of adjuvant

The World Health Organization (1990) recommends a step-like approach in the selection of pain medications which is graphically depicted above.

The stepped approach can be ineffective if the health care provider does not use clinical judgment to decide which step to start a person on when he or she has moderate to severe pain. For example, someone with pain from a compression fracture of the lower spine due to osteoprosis may be in quite severe pain, particularly if the fracture is recent. This person may need Step Three opioid pain medications in addition to other analgesics. Many experts would consider adding a fourth step to take into account many procedures such as epidural steroid injections and other surgical or anesthesia techniques that are recognized as being successful at relieving pain.

Analgesics: Dosing Changes in the Older Adult

Did you know that recommended doses of analgesics for older adults are often lower than those prescribed for younger adults? This is due to changes that affect all of us as we age. *Harrison's Principles of Internal Medicine*, the classic reference for internal medicine, explains age-related changes and their effect on drug metabolism.

Greater fat to muscle ratio. As we age, our muscles become smaller, and we also have relatively more fat in the body. Medications that are stored in fat (e.g., benzodiazepines such as diazepam and lorazepam) tend to last longer in the body, thereby causing side effects and toxicity.

Less water. There is less water in the bodies of older persons because the tissue does not hold as much as tissue in young bodies. This means that the concentration of medications in the blood and tissue is higher and may cause more side effects if doses are not adjusted.

Lower protein levels in the blood. Older adults have a greater chance of chronic illness and inadequate nutrition that may lead to lower protein levels in the blood. Some medications will bind more or less to the protein. The active drug is the part that is not bound to the protein. Most of the dose of an NSAID analgesic binds to protein in the blood, so if there is less protein, there is more active drug circulating in the individual. In seniors, for this reason these drugs tend to cause greater side effects and toxicity than in younger persons.

Slower metabolism and clearance of medications. Older adults may metabolize medications more slowly because the liver's capacity for breaking down medications for removal from the body is lower than before. The kidneys' capacity for removing the breakdown products of the drug is also slower with age. The medication therefore builds up in the blood and can cause increased side effects and toxicity.

These changes become more significant with increasing age, particularly when they occur at the same time as other medical illnesses. We tend to refer to some seniors as *frail* when such changes are profound. These people may still be living in the community but are somewhat less independent and require more medical follow-up. Thus, the doctor must first make a judgment about whether the person has the attributes of a frail elder, then change medication doses appropriately.

Classes of Pain Medication

In the sections above, we reviewed some general information about how to take pain medications. We also examined the way in which health professionals tend to make decisions about analgesics. Now, we will take a closer look at the different classes of pain medications. These include acetaminophen (paracetamol), anti-inflammatory drugs (NSAIDS), and opioids.

If you are currently taking pain medications, see if you can identify which classes they belong to. Moreover, as you read further about the drugs you take, pay close attention to the information about the mechanism of action (i.e., how the medication works), the dose, route of administration (e.g., injection, pill), side effects, drug interactions, and effectiveness. The information may be too technical for some readers, but do not be discouraged. Talk with your doctor or pharmacist about any questions you may have about your medications.

Acetaminophen (Paracetamol)

Acetaminophen (known as paracetamol in the United Kingdom) is the most commonly used non-opioid analgesic or painkiller. The most common brand is Tylenol®. This particular brand name is used interchangeably with acetaminophen, although other companies also manufacture the product. It is important to remember that acetaminophen is a different product from aspirin (acetylsalicylic acid). Aspirin is an NSAID and is used for pain associated with inflammation and also for fever. The side effects of aspirin are different from those of acetaminophen. One of the most serious aspirin side effects is a major bleed from the stomach, especially in the older person who may have had no previous warnings of stomach problems. Acetaminophen is similar to aspirin in its pain-relieving and fever-reducing effects, but it does not have the side effects of aspirin. Acetaminophen is inexpensive and available over the counter. It is usually the first line of therapy (i.e., Step one on page 152), and many individuals begin using it on their own.

Sometimes, the variety of mixtures of medications is confusing. There are numerous combinations of acetaminophen: acetaminophen with codeine or acetaminophen with codeine and caffeine, for instance. The number and amount of drugs in these preparations can vary depending on the manufacturer and the country. The same holds true with aspirin (some pain relievers contain a combination of aspirin, caffeine, and codeine). There are also various formulations of acetaminophen-type analgesics such as chewable, long-acting, and suppository forms. Check with your local pharmacist to see what is available to you. You should carefully read labels to avoid unwanted side effects.

Mechanism of action. The way acetaminophen works is not well understood. It is a strong inhibitor of cyclooxygenase, a chemical that is present when a person has a fever. In addition, it may affect pain pathways within the central nervous system. It may also alter the formation or action of chemical substances that affect pain.

Dosage range. The dose for acetaminophen is usually 2000 to 4000 mg per day, and the maximum recommended dose for persons with normal kidney and liver function is 4000 mg per day. The dose should be reduced by 50% to 75% for those with abnormal kidney or liver function, or the physician might suggest a different therapy altogether. Acetaminophen is an ingredient found in many different medications, so when determining how much you are taking, combine the amounts from all of your medications. Be sure to seek your physician's advice about the amount of medication that is best for you.

Route of administration. This medication is generally taken by mouth, there is a liquid form, as well as pills and caplets. Both plain acetaminophen (325 mg) and extra strength acetaminophen (500 mg) are available over the counter.

Side effects and their management. Side effects are rare with acetaminophen. Some individuals may experience mild stomach upset. Unusual sensitivity reactions may occur, such as rashes or hives. Overdose may lead to acute liver damage, but this is very rare in the usual therapeutic doses.

Drug interactions. Again, drug interactions are not usual with acetaminophen. Occasionally there is a rise in the INR (a lab test for blood clotting) in a person taking warfarin-type blood thinners (e.g., Coumadin®).

Effectiveness. Acetaminophen is effective for many mild types of pain, and an appropriate dose may be taken every four to six hours while you are awake to prevent pain symptoms. Long-acting formulations may last up to eight hours.

NSAIDs

There are two types of NSAIDs or nonsteroidal anti-inflammatory drugs —the older ones, which include ibuprofen, naproxen, and ketoprofen; and the newer class, such as celecoxib. Generally, NSAID therapy is used for pain control when maximum doses of acetaminophen are not working.

NSAIDs help reduce pain and inflammation that may be due to injury from a fall, infection, or degenerative conditions. It also helps control inflammation in other conditions such as osteoarthritis, though in this case there may be pain without inflammation. (Inflammation in the joints causes redness, heat, and swelling.)

There is a relatively new group of these drugs known as cyclooxygenase-2 or COX-2 agents (e.g., celecoxib). These appear to cause fewer significant gastrointestinal bleeds than the older agents (e.g., ibuprofen, naproxen), but overall there is a similar range of effectiveness and side effects for these products. Individuals may respond better to one product than to another. So, it is important to work with your doctor to find the drug(s) that are most successful for you. This new

156

class of NSAIDs is more expensive than the older class. A combination of acetaminophen and an NSAID is unlikely to provide an overall gain in pain relief. Most NSAIDs are available by prescription, although ibuprofen is also available over the counter in the United States.

Route of administration. Oral. Topical formulations of diclofenac, one of the older NSAIDS, are available in some countries.

Side effects and their management. At first, studies suggested that the newer NSAIDs were less likely to cause serious gastrointestinal side effects, such as bleeding, but questions are now being raised about this. The frequency of kidney side effects (i.e., salt and water retention and damage to kidney tissue) appears to be the same in both groups. Other side effects are possible (e.g., hypertension, increased risk of heart attack).

Effectiveness. When pain is due to active inflammation, anti-inflammatory medications are the treatment of choice. If you have kidney problems, hypertension, heart problems, or other chronic illnesses, check with your physician to make sure these drugs are safe for you.

Opioids

Opioids are strictly prescription drugs. Analgesics belonging to the opioid class are also known as narcotics, but that term has been associated with the abuse of these medications and with criminal and social problems. The term "opioid" is the true name of this class and indicates helpful pain-relieving properties that have been known for thousands of years. Before going further we need to consider many of the myths that have grown around the use of these medications and that have made many people fearful of using them.

Myths about opioids. These are the most common worries for patients or their doctors about the use of morphine and other opioids:

Patient: *"I'm getting morphine because there is nothing else to do and they have given up on me."*

"I will get addicted if I take morphine."

"If I take morphine I will die sooner."

"If I use too much morphine now it may not work when I really need it."

Doctor: *"Prescribing these medications may get me into trouble with the regulators of opioids, and I could lose my license to practice."*

Let's look at the arguments refuting these concerns:

1. **Patient: "I'm getting morphine because there is nothing else to do and they have given up on me."** This myth dates back to early times when physicians were so fearful of addiction to morphine that they waited until people were near death before prescribing it. Many people suffered terrible pain because of the reluctance to use these medications. We now know that morphine and other opioids can be used at any time to manage pain. If the pain can be controlled through another treatment, then the morphine can be stopped.

2. **Patient: "I will get addicted if I take morphine."** Because of the fear of addiction, these medications became illegal without a prescription, in the early 1900s. In those times, everyone who took opioids for more than a few weeks was considered an addict. Now pain researchers estimate that only 2% to 5% of all patients with chronic pain have a true addiction. Unfortunately, undertreated, debilitating pain is much more common. Addiction as we now understand it is more about the person than the medication. But yes, you may become dependent on your morphine for pain control, just as a diabetic is dependent on insulin to control blood sugars.

We now view addiction as the "Four C's":

- ◉ *Compulsive use*
- ◉ *Loss of Control*
- ◉ *Craving for the drug*
- ◉ *Use despite bad Consequences*

People who have the disposition to have addiction will find themselves using increasing amounts of the drug, unable to reduce the dose, obtaining the drug illegally, and using it despite bad consequences (worse pain control, family distress over their behavior, etc.). They may not be taking the medication for pain, but rather for an escape from their life.

Someone who uses opioids for pain on a regular basis will develop what is called physical dependence, which means the body notices if

158

the medication suddenly is withdrawn. This used to be called *withdrawal* and is characterized by tremors, insomnia, diarrhea, or agitation. We now know that this is not necessarily a sign of addiction but shows that the body's previous adaptation must be considered when the medication is withdrawn.

3. *Patient: "If I take morphine I will die sooner."* Again, this myth arose because morphine was used only in the last day or so of life because of fear and ignorance about its properties. We now know that morphine is a safe drug if used appropriately in people with pain or shortness of breath. Drs. Thomas and von Gunten, palliative care physicians and researchers, have pointed out that there are now multiple studies looking at the opioids and sedatives that are used in end-of-life care and that these medications do not shorten life. In fact, some research suggests that cancer patients who have good pain relief may live longer. Pain is a stress on the body and, if unrelieved, it may make the body sicker.

4. *Patient: "If I use too much morphine now it may not work when I really need it."* Some people require small doses to control their pain while others need large doses. Each person is different, and there is no maximum dose of opioids. Rather, we concentrate on what dose relieves pain with the fewest side effects. In the face of stable disease, tolerance—increased doses need to get effective pain relief—is very slow to develop. If you or your doctor observe a significant need for more opioids to control pain, you should have a medical assessment for a new or progressive disease.

5. *Doctor: "Prescribing these medications may get me into trouble with the regulators of opioids, and I could lose my license to practice."* Physicians must have adequate education and experience in prescribing opioids appropriately. A specific diagnosis and a rational treatment plan ensure that opioid prescriptions for acute and chronic pain syndromes are suitable for the patient. Adequate follow-up and ongoing monitoring are important in order to optimize the treatment and improve the quality of life of the pain patient. Doctors who follow these basic guidelines do not need to fear regulators.

Route of administration. Opioids can be administered in various formulations, which gives them great flexibility. Often, they are given as oral medications—pills or liquid—which is most convenient and least expensive. However, opioids are also available in suppositories and injectable forms. These are used when the person cannot swallow. One opioid comes as a patch that is placed on the skin and releases a constant small dose into the patient's bloodstream. The route of administration depends on many factors, including the ability to swallow, the side effects, the type of opioid best suited to the person, and convenience.

Side effects. Common side effects include constipation, dry mouth, drowsiness, and sweating. Less common side effects include bad dreams, hallucinations, confusion, muscle jerking, itching, bladder dysfunction, and respiratory depression. Here are some key points about side effects:

- Used appropriately, opioids have no long-term permanent side effects, which means they are safer than many other medications we use.

- There is no damage to the organs with regular use of opioids.

- Everyone who uses opioids gets constipated. **Constipation** does not go away if you take the medication on a regular basis. A stimulant laxative is necessary. Stimulants such as senna, cascara, glycerine or bisacodyl, combined with a stool softener such as docusate, are best. Lactulose can be added if the former combinations do not work adequately.

- **Nausea** is common when a patient first takes opioids but will often resolve after the first week. If the person has been nauseated by other opioids in the past, it is best to take an antinausea medication for the first week or two. The best medications to take for nausea related to opioids are prescription medications called metoclopramide and domperidone rather than dimenhydrinate (Dramamine® or Gravol®).

- **Dry mouth** is very common. Sucking on sugar-free candies can help, as can using an artificial saliva spray available over the counter.

- **Sleepiness or sedation** occurs during the first few days of starting an opioid or increasing the dose. After that, you should not feel any added drowsiness. If sedation persists after five days, your health care provider should be informed.

- **Hallucinations and bad dreams** after opioid use are not a sign of mental instability and should be reported to your health care professional. When these side effects do occur, a different opioid should be used.

- **Confusion** is very disturbing and should also be reported. If the right opioid is used in the correct dose, the person should expect to be alert and able to carry on normally.

- **Itching** is not a sign of allergy unless there are hives (red welts) on the skin. Itching will often resolve over the first few weeks, and a nonsedating antihistamine will help during this period.

- **Muscle jerking** may mean that the dose of the opioid is too high or is not the right one for the patient. A few twitches are common, but if they become frequent and interfere with activity, they should be reported.

- **The inability to empty the bladder** completely is an uncommon side effect seen in the first few days of use of opioids. The problem usually disappears.

- **Respiratory depression** is the slowing of the respiratory system due to opioids. This is only significant if a person first using opioids is given too large a dose. When taking opioids regularly, the body rapidly adapts to this effect, and changes in the dose can be made without any significant effect on the respiratory system.

Effectiveness. Opioids can be extremely effective at relieving pain, particularly pain from cancer, arthritis, degenerative changes in the spine, osteoporosis fractures, and other painful conditions. It may take a patient, working with the doctor, several weeks to choose the right opioid and to adjust the dose in order to achieve the best pain relief with the fewest side effects.

It is possible that you did not see one of your pain medications in the classes of analgesics presented above. Don't worry! In addition to the different classes of analgesics presented above, there are other types of medications that doctors may use to manage your pain. Most of these are described in the next section.

Other Medications and Therapies

Physicians also prescribe highly effective drugs known as *coanalgesics* or *adjuvant* pain medications. Most adjuvant analgesics are used in neuropathic pain (e.g., pain from shingles or poststroke pain) resulting from damage to a nerve or to the spinal cord and brain. Neuropathic pain can often persist long after the damage has healed and can respond poorly to regular analgesics such as acetaminophen, NSAIDs, or opioid-type drugs.

Adjuvant medications often do not work immediately the way that regular analgesics do. Often they function by reducing the sensitivity of a damaged nerve or by increasing the pain threshold of the patient. It is important to take these medications as directed even though they may not seem to help the pain right away. The dosage of these drugs varies widely and must be individually adjusted according to the effectiveness of the medications and their side effects. As a rule, the best dose is the one that achieves the most pain relief with the fewest side effects.

Adjuvants are medications originally developed to treat certain disorders but which have been discovered, as a side-light, to provide effective relief for other unrelated conditions as well. Therefore, they often have names referring to those other diseases that they were originally intended to treat. Here are some examples (using generic drug names):

> *Tricyclic antidepressants: amitriptyline, nortriptyline, desipramine*
>
> *Other antidepressants: venlafaxine, mirtazapine, paroxetine*
>
> *Anticonvulsants: gabapentin, carbamazepine, topiramate*
>
> *Steroid medications: prednisone, dexamethasone*
>
> *Bisphosphonates: clodronate, pamidronate*

Topical medications have also been developed for use either in neuropathic pain or pain that is close to the surface of the body. *Topical* means that the medication is in a cream which is rubbed on the body where pain is present. Topical NSAIDs have been proven effective in treating inflamed joints. Topical local anesthetics have been used to relieve painful damaged nerves near the surface such as in postherpetic neuralgia (pain that persists after shingles).

In addition to the above, anesthesia interventions represent another form of drug treatment. For local pain, an injection of anesthetic may be helpful but not long-lasting in many cases. In some pain clinics, anesthetists are part of teams devoted to pain relief. Their expertise is used to provide treatment of specific pain syndromes.

Future Directions in Pain Management

New medications are always being developed, but almost all of the pain that people experience can be treated effectively with the techniques and medications we have today. The importance of fostering a sense of teamwork among the affected person, the doctor, other health profession-als, and family members is crucial to ongoing assessment of pain and to the way the pain responds to the medication and other treatments.

Common Pain-Related Conditions Among Seniors

In addition to learning more about pain medications, you might find it helpful to review the types of pain-related conditions that are widespread among seniors. Chronic medical conditions become more prevalent with increasing age. Many of these problems involve pain.

In the United States, most older adults who take pain medications tend to have diagnoses of arthritis (44%), bone and joint pain (31%), and low back pain (16%). A description of these and other common pain condi-tions is provided below.

If you are an older adult, it is likely that you, or someone you know, may experience one or more of the following conditions:

- *Arthritis/rheumatism*
- *Back problems (nonarthritic) such as spinal stenosis or osteoporosis*
- *Stomach/intestinal disorders (e.g., gastric reflux disease, hiatus hernia, diverticular diseases)*

- *Chronic bronchitis/emphysema*
- *Cancer pain*
- *Heart disease (e.g., angina)*
- *Neuropathic pain conditions*

Arthritis

The term *arthritis* refers to problems involving the joint and the ligaments, tendons, or muscles around the joint. According to Kate Lorig and James F. Fries, two arthritis experts, there are over 120 different kinds of arthritis that involve different joints in the body. Common types of arthritis include osteoarthritis, rheumatoid arthritis, and gout.

Osteoarthritis (also referred to as *degenerative joint disease*) usually affects the joints in the hands, knees, and hips and develops as a result of years of normal wear and tear. Individuals with osteoarthritis typically report deep, aching pain in one or more joints. The probability of developing osteoarthritis increases as we age.

Rheumatoid arthritis is less common and occurs when the body's immune system begins to attack the tissues that line the inside of the joint. This condition involves aching joint pain and is associated with morning stiffness, swelling, and pain or tenderness with motion at one or more joints. The cause of rheumatoid arthritis is unknown at this time.

Gout is an acute form of arthritis that results in flareups of aching, sharp, throbbing pain. It commonly affects the ankles and feet (especially the big toe) and occurs when uric acid accumulates in the joint.

Rheumatism

The term *rheumatism* does not refer to a specific disease or disorder. Rather, it is a term that is used in a general way to describe pain and stiffness in the muscles and joints. It is broadly used to describe conditions such as osteoarthritis, rheumatoid arthritis, and other pain-related problems such as bursitis, lumbago (i.e., low back pain), tendonitis, and sciatica.

Back Pain

Back pain may occur at any point from the neck to the tailbone. The pain may be restricted to a specific area or be diffuse (i.e., spread out). Back pain can have many causes including muscle strain or mechanical problems, infection, trauma, inflammatory rheumatological disorders (rheumatoid arthritis), Paget's disease (defined below), and cancer. Some of the more common conditions that lead to back pain among older adults are briefly described below.

Spinal stenosis. This condition usually occurs with advancing age and involves a narrowing of the spinal canal. The narrowing creates pressure on the spinal nerves which may be associated with back and leg pain. Drs. Merskey and Bogduk, two distinguished pain researchers, say that the pain may be experienced as a numb, heavy feeling extending from the buttock to the foot. This condition occurs as our bodies age and is seen mostly in patients over the age of 50.

Paget's disease involves the abnormal formation of bone tissue resulting in weakened and deformed bones. Pain is the most common symptom of this disease and can affect any bone (not just the back).

Degenerative disk disease occurs when the disks in the spine begin to wear out. This narrows the space between the vertebrae and compresses the nerves, resulting in pain.

Sciatica is associated with pain that radiates from the lower back down through the legs. Pain occurs when the sciatic nerve, which exits the spinal cord at the end of the lumbar spine, is compressed or irritated.

Osteoporosis. This disorder occurs when the bones lose calcium, causing them to become fragile and prone to breaking. This disease is more common among women than men and can lead to painful back problems. Its negative consequences are not limited to the back and can affect other parts of the body.

Slipped disk (degenerative spondylolisthesis). This condition occurs when a vertebra slips forward or sideways out of position and presses an adjacent nerve root onto the one below it. This frequently occurs in the lower back (i.e., the *lumbar* region). Individuals with a slipped disk commonly report pain or tenderness in the area where the slip has occurred. When a disk moves out of position, discomfort may also be reported in the thighs and buttocks. If pressure is exerted on the nerve roots, leg weakness or numbness may occur along with pain that radiates down the legs.

Stomach Ulcers

Ulcers or inflammation may occur in the lining of the stomach and, if left untreated, may produce chronic pain. Stomach ulcers may occur at any age, but they are most common among middle-aged and elderly individuals. Pain usually occurs after a meal and is localized over the upper or middle part of the abdomen. Diagnosis of ulcers is very important because certain types can be treated with antibiotics.

Chronic Bronchitis/Emphysema

Certain respiratory problems may be associated with chronic pain among older adults as the physical act of breathing becomes difficult.

Bronchitis is a disease in which the bronchial tubes (i.e., the airways that extend from the windpipe to the lungs) become swollen and inflamed. As a result, the bronchial tubes produce mucus. Excess mucus usually triggers a persistent cough. Together the inflammation and mucus make it difficult for the individual to breathe.

Emphysema occurs when the tiny air sacs in the lungs (called "alveoli") are damaged. The lungs begin to lose their elasticity, and normal air exchange is impaired (air exchange means that carbon dioxide is exhaled while oxygen is inhaled). When active, individuals with emphysema may become short of breath and experience wheezing, coughing, and chest tightness.

Cancer Pain

The term *cancer* refers to abnormal cell growth that destroys healthy tissue in the body. As cancerous cells multiply, they may form a mass or tumor. It is possible for cancer cells to spread to other parts of the body (i.e., metastasize), where they invade and destroy other healthy tissue.

Older adults are more likely than any other age group to suffer from cancer. Among older men, common types of cancer include prostate, lung, and colorectal cancer. Among older women, common cancer diagnoses include breast, lung, and colorectal cancer. The treatment of cancer may also produce pain. Surgical procedures, bone marrow biopsies, chemotherapy, radiation, and even lengthy X-ray procedures may cause discomfort over and above the pain associated with the cancer and any other preexisting, long-term conditions.

Heart Disease

Older adults have a higher rate of heart disease than any other age group. When blood vessels around the heart (coronary arteries) become narrow, less blood and oxygen reach the heart muscle. Chest pain (angina pectoris) and heart attack (myocardial infarction) may occur. Heart disease may involve abnormal heart rhythms (such as atrial fibrillation). Advanced heart disease may lead to congestive heart failure. This diagnosis is given when the heart has difficulty pumping blood, leading to the collection of blood in the lungs and other parts of the body.

Neuropathic Pain Conditions

These disorders arise in response to problems within the peripheral or central nervous systems (e.g., shingles or pain following a stroke). Neuropathic pain is commonly described as burning, tingling, or shooting pain. This type of pain may not respond to stronger opioids as well as other types of pain, or very high doses may be required. Two of these conditions are described below.

Postherpetic neuralgia is one form of chronic neuropathic pain that usually follows a case of shingles. Individuals suffering from shingles (or "herpes zoster") experience a painful rash that spreads along an area served by one or two sensory nerves. These nerves, commonly thoracic, extend from the back around the individual's rib cage on one side of the body. Pain that persists once the rash goes away is diagnosed as postherpetic neuralgia.

Poststroke pain is another form of neuropathic pain. It is also referred to as *central poststroke pain,* formerly called *thalamic pain.* As the name implies, this condition is associated with pain that occurs because of damage to the nervous system following a stroke. Described as burning, aching, or lancinating, the pain may occur shortly after the stroke happens, or it may begin several months later.

Summary

We hope that by reading this chapter you have gained a better understanding of how medications may be used most effectively to manage pain (e.g., scheduling the timing of medications to produce continuous pain relief). Further, we hope that this chapter will serve as a basic reference guide about medications and pain conditions. If you have any additional questions after reading this chapter, talk to your doctor. After all, it's your right to be well informed!

THOMAS HADJISTAVROPOULOS, PHD, RD PSYCH.
RONALD R. MARTIN, PHD, RD PSYCH.

CHAPTER ELEVEN

Information for Caregivers of Older Adults Who Have Dementia

Very often, older adults as well as their friends and relatives care for a frail loved one who suffers from pain. Caring for older adults who have dementia (e.g., Alzheimer's disease) is especially common. There are distinctive challenges that are common to seniors with dementia. As dementia progresses, the ability to communicate verbally deteriorates. As a result, people with dementia may not be able to tell others about their pain (e.g., that they have pain, where they feel it, and whether it is getting better or worse). Many patients with dementia tend to become aggressive when they have pain and, as a result, are often prescribed psychiatric medications instead of painkillers. Pain among people with dementia is often undertreated because it is often not recognized. As a result, many older persons not only suffer from pain but also feel helpless and become depressed. It is, therefore, important to recognize pain in this population.

Recognizing Pain

Older adults with mild to moderate dementia are usually able to tell others that they have pain and can point to the painful area. However, the ability to report pain deteriorates as the dementia becomes more severe. Because many older adults with dementia tend not to report pain as often, we sometimes have to rely on recognizing behaviors that may indicate the presence of pain. Such behaviors include facial expressions (e.g., grimaces), tense muscles, fidgeting, screaming, moaning, noisy breathing, agitation, difficulty sleeping, sweating, and refusing care.

At the end of this chapter, you will find a checklist called the Pain Assessment Checklist for Seniors with Limited Ability to Communicate (PACSLAC). The PACSLAC can help you recognize signs of pain in a loved one. We recommend that caregivers who are concerned about pain in a loved one with dementia complete the PACSLAC regularly. For the most effective results, it is best to observe the loved one under consistent circumstances. You could, for example, complete the checklist during personal care or over the course of an evening. Choose one situation or the other, but do not compare PACSLAC behaviors across different situations. You should not compare a score based on observations during personal care to one based on observations made throughout an evening. Personal care monitoring should be compared to similar situations that also involve the same activities.

The PACSLAC is scored by summing up all of the items. It is best to use this checklist in an individualized way. That is, fill it out regularly while observing your loved one, even when pain is not suspected. If the scores increase suddenly, pain could well be present. It is important to record the scores over time (in a diary such as the one provided at the end of this chapter).

However, the PACSLAC is not a definitive indicator of pain. That is, sometimes it may fail to identify pain, and other times it may suggest that pain is present when in fact it is not. In addition to regular medical checkups, it is always important to consult with a doctor when you suspect that your loved one may be experiencing pain. *Moreover, it is important to remember that factors other than pain (e.g., being upset about something) can also increase scores on the PACSLAC. For this reason any conclusions based on use of the PACSLAC should be considered tentative. Please consult with your loved one's doctor if you are using the PACSLAC.*

If the doctor needs more information about the PACSLAC, there are scientific articles that he or she can read to learn more about it, for example, the articles by Fuchs-Lacelle and Hadjistavropoulos (2004) as well as Zwakhalen et al. (2006) in the bibliography at the end of the book. Research on the PACSLAC is continuing. Please refer to the disclaimer in the opening pages of this volume.

Managing Pain

In addition to a variety of medications and treatments (prescribed by a doctor or other health professional), other factors might help your loved one prevent and manage pain.

Exercise. *In Aging, Physical Activity and Health,* R.J. Shephard states, *"There is no known pharmacological remedy that can safely and effectively reduce a person's biological age and enhance his or her quality adjusted life-expectancy. Regular physical activity has the potential to do this and more."* Exercise is also an effective way to lessen chronic pain. Research has also led to the conclusion that higher levels of physical activity can have a positive effect on cognitive functioning. It is essential that older adults check with a doctor or other qualified health professional before starting any exercise program since exercise might worsen some conditions (e.g., certain heart ailments) and may involve certain risks (e.g., falls).

An exercise consultation should always be conducted where frail seniors are involved, but older adults with dementia can often benefit from an appropriately designed exercise program (e.g., a physiotherapist-supervised passive range-of-motion program that could reduce stiffness).

Pleasant activities. Pleasant activities can help improve a patient's quality of life and distract him or her from pain. Because you know your loved one best, you may be aware of activities that he or she enjoys (e.g., going for a short walk, listening to music, spending time with pets). Regularly taking part in such activities, and increasing their frequency, will probably improve your loved one's mood and ability to cope with pain. According to an American Psychiatric Association document, research provides modest support for the idea that pet therapy and other environmental interventions improve function and mood among patients with dementia. Here are some steps that you could follow:

◎ Make a list of your loved one's preferred activities. Contact other relatives and friends who might provide additional pleasant activities for the list.

◎ At first, it may be difficult to initiate certain pleasant activities in your loved one's routine. Provide emotional and physical support and be patient. Over time, increase your loved one's participation in these activities.

◎ Reduce sources of negative behaviors and increase positive interactions. Pain-related and other negative behaviors (e.g., complaints, agitation) may be very likely even when your loved one is engaging in pleasant activities. When these behaviors occur, try to keep track of what happens before, during, and after. This may help you identify the source of the negative behavior. Try using the Pain Behavior Data Sheet provided at the end of the chapter. Sometimes, negative behaviors result from a dislike for a specific part of the pleasant activity (e.g., setting up a board game). They may also be triggered by certain people or objects, or by noises and other distractions. You may be able to eliminate certain triggers (e.g., in some circumstances you may be able to reduce noise levels). We also recommend that the caregiver makes a special effort to interact more with, and pay more attention to, the loved one when he or she is calm and interacts well. This should increase the frequency of positive interactions. These interactions could also be encouraged with verbal praise, nonverbal encouragement (e.g., smiling at the person you care for), and favorite activities over and above those that would normally occur.

Consultation with a physiotherapist. A physiotherapist or other qualified health professional may be able to assess your loved one not only with respect to appropriate exercise but with other activities that could improve the ability to function. For example, for a patient who has difficulty using his or her hands, larger utensils are generally easier to handle than smaller ones and are available in a variety of places. A physiotherapist could also help you with recommendations about a loved one who is restricted to a bed or a wheelchair and might need to be properly positioned and repositioned in order to avoid stiffness.

Take Care of Yourself

Caring for a loved can have many benefits for the caregiver. A study from the University of Toronto has shown that most caregivers identify positive aspects in the caregiving experience. At the same time, it is very common for caregivers to feel depressed or overwhelmed with the caregiving role. Caregivers must make sure to protect their own health and take care of their own needs. This will ensure that they do a better job helping their loved ones.

A variety of resources are available to assist family caregivers. These range from daycare services for seniors who suffer from dementia to part-time home nursing care. These resources also include full residential care for seniors with severe problems who require around-the-clock professional care. Many countries now have support groups and other services for caregivers (sources of relevant information are listed at the end of this chapter). Social support helps all caregivers maintain their own physical and emotional well-being and in addition allows them to provide better-quality care for their loved ones.

Summary

Patients with dementia (e.g., Alzheimer's disease) often suffer from pain problems. While patients with mild to moderate dementia can usually tell others that they are in pain, the signs that they are experiencing discomfort become more difficult to recognize as the dementia progresses. This chapter provides information about a specific method (the PACSLAC) designed to help caregivers recognize signs of pain, but this method does not represent a definitive indicator. That is, sometimes this method may fail to identify pain, and other times it may suggest that pain is present when in fact it is not. In addition to regular medical checkups, consult with a doctor when you suspect that your loved one may be experiencing physical distress. A physiotherapist will typically be able to design a safe exercise program that can help prevent pain. Engaging the person with dementia in pleasant activities will often help distract him or her from pain and improve quality of life. At the same time, we recognize that caring for a loved one with dementia can be a demanding task. Joining a caregiver support group in your community can be an enormous help. It is very important that caregivers do everything they can to take care of themselves and their needs, because when caregivers feel better, they provide better care.

Pain Assessment Checklist for Seniors with Limited Ability to Communicate (PACSLAC)

Date: _____ Time Assessed: _____

Name of Patient/Resident: _____

Purpose: This checklist is used to assess pain in persons who have dementia and are unable to communicate verbally.

Instructions: Indicate with a checkmark which of the items on the PACSLAC occurred at least once during the period of interest. Use only one check mark per item. Even if an item (e.g., *grimacing*) occurs more than once, it should only receive one checkmark.

To generate a Total Pain Score, add up the total number of check marks (the maximum score is 60, but most patients with pain obtain much lower scores).

This chapter describes how the PACSLAC could be used.

Comments:

_____

_____

_____

_____

_____

_____

Pain Assessment Checklist continued...

Facial Expressions		Uncooperative/resistant to care	
Grimacing		Guarding sore area	
Sad look		Touching/holding sore area	
Tight face		Limping	
Dirty look		Clenched fist	
Change in eyes (e.g., squinting, dull, bright, increased movement)		Going into fetal position	
		Stiffness/rigidity	
Frowning		**Social/Personality/Mood**	
Pained expression		Physical aggression (e.g., pushing people and/or objects, scratching others, hitting others, striking, kicking)	
Grim face			
Clenching teeth		Verbal aggression	
Wincing		Not wanting to be touched	
Opening mouth		Not allowing people near	
Creasing forehead		Angry/mad	
Screwing up nose		Throwing things	
Activity/Body Movement		Increased confusion	
Fidgeting		Anxious	
Pulling away		Upset	
Flinching		Agitated	
Restlessness		Cranky/irritable	
Pacing		Frustrated	
Wandering		Other*	
Trying to leave		Pale face	
Refusing to move		Flushed, red face	
Thrashing		Teary eyed	
Decreased activity		Sweating	
Refusing medications		Shaking/trembling	
Moving slowly		Skin cold, clammy	
Impulsive behavior (e.g., repetitive movements)		Changes in sleep (please circle): Decreased sleep Increased sleep during day	

176

Pain Assessment Checklist continued...

Changes in appetite (please circle):
   Decreased appetite
   Increased appetite
		Grunting	

		Subscale Scores	
Screaming/yelling		Facial expressions	
Calling out (i.e., for help)		Activity/body movement	
Crying		Social/personality/mood	
Specific sound or vocalization for pain (e.g., "ow," "ouch")		Other*	
		Total Checklist Score	
Moaning and groaning		** Other subscale includes physiological changes, eating and sleeping changes, and vocal behaviors.*	
Mumbling			

Please note that the PACSLAC is not a definitive indicator of pain. That is, sometimes it may fail to identify pain and other times it may suggest that pain is present when in fact it is not. In addition to regular medical checkups, it is always important to consult with a doctor when you suspect that your loved one may be experiencing pain. If the doctor needs more information about the PACSLAC, there are scientific articles that he or she can read to learn more about it (see, for example, Fuchs-Lacelle and Hadjistavropoulos 2004 as well as Zwakhalen et al. 2006 in the bibliography at the end of the book).

The PACSLAC is copyrighted © by Shannon Fuchs-Lacelle and Thomas Hadjistavropoulos and is reproduced here with permission. Individuals who have purchased this book may make copies of the PACSLAC for their personal use.

PACSLAC Diary Sheet

Be sure to read the instructions about the PACSLAC in this chapter prior to completing this sheet. Feel free to make copies of this page for your personal use.

Date/Time	Situation (e.g., while assisting my loved one to move from his/her chair to bed)	PACSLAC Score

Pain Behavior Data Sheet

You may complete this form after you have observed your loved one's pain behavior or other negative behavior. The purpose of this form is to help identify the sources and consequences of his or her pain behavior or other negative behavior. Feel free to make copies of this sheet for your personal use.

Date/Time	Description of pain-related behavior (frequency, intensity, duration) (e.g., grimacing)	What happened just before the pain behavior? (e.g., medical procedures, adverse events, behaviors, mood states, people, places, things)	What were the consequences of the pain behavior? (e.g., avoiding, escaping)	What may have caused the pain?	Recommendations (if any) to prevent future pain?	Comment on the effectiveness of intervention, if used (note changes in duration, frequency, intensity of pain)
3 / 21/ 07 10:30 a.m.	He was agitated and began to yell. Happened four times (10 minutes each time). Moderate intensity.	Sitting in wheelchair, leaning to one side, alone in his room.	Responded to him (talking, providing snacks). Resident repositioned.	Pressure sore sitting in one position?	Reposition patient regularly.	Patient stopped yelling. Less agitation.

Resources for Caregivers

Alzheimer's associations in various countries offer information for caregivers. Many of these associations also offer caregiver support groups. For information, contact the Alzheimer's association in your country.

Australia:
Website: http://www.alzheimers.org.au
Telephone: +61 02 6254 4233

Canada:
Website: http://www.alzheimer.ca
Telephone (toll free): 1-800-616-8816

New Zealand:
Website: http://www.alzheimers.org.nz
Telephone: +64 04 381 2362

United Kingdom:
Website: http://www.alzheimers.org.uk
Telephone: +44 020 7306 0606

United States:
Website: http://www.alz.org
Telephone (toll-free 24-hour help line): 1-800-272-3900

Final Thoughts

In this book, you have been exposed to information about pain among seniors and strategies for managing pain in adaptive ways. A variety of related topics were addressed in this pain management program including psychological means for coping with pain, mood, social support and loneliness, physical activity, ergonomics, medications, sleep hygiene, nutrition, and effective communication with health care providers.

In learning about these pain management topics, you may have come across certain subjects or treatment strategies that were somewhat difficult for you to master. Keep in mind that this is natural when learning something new. For example, if you were learning to play the piano, you might find certain skills easy to master (e.g., playing scales) whereas others are more difficult (e.g., "sight reading" music). The key to learning new things is to "stick with it." With time and regular practice, things that take effort at first become easier and more automatic. The same is true for your pain management skills.

The material in this book requires patience and practice but can result in effective pain management. Dealing more effectively with pain means better quality of life for you and, indirectly, for those you care about. So, you owe it to yourself to maintain and increase the skills that help you take care of your pain.

Although people usually feel better once they begin to use their pain management skills, it is not uncommon for pain-related problems to worsen occasionally. Remember, setbacks such as this are common among those who strive to manage their chronic pain in better ways. In fact, one could argue that continuing to use your pain management skills is crucial when such situations arise, because you will most likely increase your chances of getting back to your normal level of functioning.

A worsening of your pain could have an impact on the way you think, feel, and behave. By paying attention to your thoughts, feelings, and actions, you may be able to tell when your pain is about to worsen and take steps to slow or prevent any further deterioration of your condition. Take a moment to consider some of the thoughts, feelings, and behaviors that signal a worsening of your pain:

> **Thoughts.** You may notice that your thought patterns change when your pain begins to get worse. Some people begin to think in "black and white" terms about their pain, or they think the worst:
>
> *"I can't do anything when I'm experiencing pain."*
>
> *"If I try to do anything I'll probably end up in the hospital."*
>
> **Feelings.** Sometimes when pain worsens, your mood changes. You begin to feel depressed or become more irritable.
>
> **Behaviors.** You may recognize that you act differently when your pain worsens. Some people isolate themselves or stop doing activities they normally find enjoyable.

If you notice that your pain is worsening, work on your coping self-statements by reviewing the section *Examining Your Thoughts* in Chapter 4 (pages 48–49) and continue to practice the relaxation techniques. Pace your activities as outlined in this book in order to maximize your ability to function. Moreover, try to maintain or improve your mood by continuing to engage in activities you find enjoyable (to the best of your abilities, given your pain) and keep your doctor informed about your condition.

It was a pleasure for us to prepare this book. We hope you learned a good deal about the management of chronic pain and that you will continue to use your pain management skills!

Please take a moment to review your progress by completing the questions on the next pages.

Pain Management Review

The best way to keep on top of your chronic pain is to be aware of the signs that tell you that you need to ramp up your use of pain management strategies.

1. List any maladaptive thoughts you may have when your pain worsens:

   _____

   _____

   _____

2. What are the emotional signs that accompany a potential worsening of pain for you?

   _____

   _____

   _____

3. What are the behavioral signs that your pain is increasing?

   _____

   _____

   _____

Pain Management Review, continued

4. Check off those areas in which you feel you have improved by using techniques described in this manual.

      ○ *More energy*

      ○ *Improved movement*

      ○ *Improved activity*

      ○ *Greater independence (e.g., being able to go shopping and do some cooking and housework)*

      ○ *Feeling more "in charge" of your life*

      ○ *Improved sleep*

      ○ *Better appetite*

      ○ *More satisfying relationships (e.g., being able to spend more "pain-free" time with others)*

      ○ *Better concentration*

      ○ *Improved mood (feeling happier and more positive)*

      ○ *Better communication with health care providers*

5. Which strategies have you found to be helpful to you? Check those that apply.

      ○ *Improving my understanding of pain*

      ○ *Increasing my social contacts*

      ○ *Distraction*

      ○ *Improving my relationships*

      ○ *Deep breathing*

      ○ *Scheduling pleasant activities*

      ○ *Relaxation*

      ○ *Pacing activities*

      ○ *Imagery*

Pain Management Review, *continued*

○ *Aerobic activity*

○ *Stretching*

○ *Identifying and changing thoughts about pain*

○ *Improving my mood*

○ *Strengthening my body*

○ *Improving my communication with my health care provider*

○ *Improving my understanding of medication*

○ *Modifying how I do things*

○ *Modifying my home environment*

6. Which chapters do I need to review?

○ **Chapter 1:** Pain among Seniors

○ **Chapter 2:** Pain and Psychology

○ **Chapter 3:** Taking Control: Effective Pain Management

○ **Chapter 4:** Pain and Emotion

○ **Chapter 5:** Social Support, Loneliness, and Pain

○ **Chapter 6:** The Role of Exercise in Seniors' Lives

○ **Chapter 7:** Living in More Comfort: Maximizing Function and Energy

○ **Chapter 8:** Sleep Hygiene and Nutrition

○ **Chapter 9:** Effective Communication with Your Doctor

○ **Chapter 10:** The Role of Medications

○ **Chapter 11:** Information for Caregivers of Older Adults who Have Dementia

Pain Management Resources from Around the World

The information from the following websites should not be used as a substitute for medical advice, diagnosis, or treatment from a qualified health professional.

When visiting some websites, you will need to find and click on links that refer to *patients, resources,* or *publications* to access information that is available to laypersons who want more information about pain.

Australia

Arthritis Australia
GPO Box 121
Sydney, NSW 2001
Australia
Phone: +61 02 9552 6085
Fax: +61 02 9552 6078
arthritisaustralia.com.au

Australian Pain Society
Dc Conferences Pty Ltd
PO Box 637
North Sydney, NSW 2059
Australia
Phone: +61 02 9954 4400
Fax: +61 02 9954 0666
www.apsoc.org.au

Australian Psychological Society
PO Box 38, Flinders Lane
Melbourne, VIC 8009
Australia
Phone: +61 03 8662 3300
Fax: +61 03 9663 6177
www.psychology.org.au

The Cancer Council Australia
GPO Box 4708
Sydney, NSW 2001
Australia
Phone: +61 02 9036 3100
Fax: +61 02 9036 3101
www.cancer.org.au

Canada

The Arthritis Society
393 University Avenue, Suite 1700
Toronto, ON
Canada M5G 1E6
Phone: 1-416-979-7228
Fax: 1-416-979-8366
www.arthritis.ca

Canadian Cancer Society
Suite 200, 10 Alcorn Avenue
Toronto, ON
Canada M4V 3B1
Phone: 1-416-961-7223
Fax: 1-416-961-4189
www.cancer.ca

Chronic Pain Association of Canada

PO Box 66017
Heritage Postal Station
#130 2323-111 Street
Edmonton, AB
Canada T6J 6T4
Phone: 1-780-482-6727
Fax: 1-780-433-3128
www.chronicpaincanada.com

The Canadian Psychological Association

141 Laurier Avenue West, Suite 702
Ottawa, ON
Canada K1P 5J3
Phone: 1-613-237-2144
Fax: 1-613-237-1674
www.cpa.ca

The Canadian Psychological Association Fact Sheet on Pain Among Seniors

www.cpa.ca/publications/
yourhealthpsychologyworksfactsheets/
chronicpainamongseniors/

Fibromyalgia-Chronic Fatigue Syndrome Canada

99 Fifth Avenue, Suite 412
Ottawa, ON
Canada K1S 5P5
http://fm-cfs.ca

New Zealand

Arthritis New Zealand

Level 2
166 Featherston Street
PO Box 10-020
Wellington
New Zealand
Phone: +64 04 472 1427
Fax: +64 04 472 7066
www.arthritis.org.nz

Cancer Society of New Zealand

PO Box 10847
Wellington 6143
New Zealand
Phone: +64 04 494 7270
Fax: +64 04 494 7271
www.cancernz.org.nz

New Zealand Pain Society

PO Box 5303
Wellington
New Zealand
www.nzps.org.nz

United Kingdom

Arthritis Care

18 Stephenson Way
London NW1 2HD
United Kingdom
Phone: +44 020 7380 6500
www.arthritiscare.org.uk

British Pain Society

Third Floor
Churchill House
35 Red Lion Square
London WC1R 4SG
United Kingdom
Phone: +44 020 7269 7840
Fax: +44 020 7831 0859
www.britishpainsociety.org

Cancerbackup

3 Bath Place
Rivington Street
London
EC2A 3JR
United Kingdom
Phone: +44 020-7696-9003
Fax: +44 020 7696 9002
www.cancerbackup.org.uk

Cancer Research UK
PO Box 123
Lincoln's Inn Fields
London WC2A 3PX
United Kingdom
Phone (Support Services):
   +44 020 7121 6699
Phone (Switchboard): +44 020 7242 0200
Fax: +44 020 7269 3100
www.cancerresearchuk.org

Fibromyalgia Association UK
PO Box 206 Stourbridge DY9 8YL
United Kingdom
Fax: +44 0870 752 5118
www.fibromyalgia-associationuk.org

United States

American Academy
of Pain Management
3947 Mono Way #A
Sonora, CA 95370
USA
Phone: 1-209-533-9744
Fax: 1-209-533-9750
www.aapainmanage.org

American Cancer Society
PO Box 22718
Oklahoma City, OK 73123-1718
USA
Phone: 1-800-ACS-2345
www.cancer.org

American Chronic Pain Association
PO Box 850
Rocklin, CA 95677
USA
Phone: 1-800-533-3231
Fax: 1-916-632-3208
www.theacpa.org

American Fibromyalgia
Syndrome Association
6380 E. Tanque Verde Road
Suite D
Tuscon, AZ 85715
USA
Phone: 1-520-733-1570
Fax: 1-520-290-5550
www.afsafund.org

American Pain Foundation
201 N Charles Street, Suite 710
Baltimore, MD 21201
USA
Phone: 1-888-615-7246
Fax: 1-410-385-1832
www.painfoundation.org

American Pain Society
4700 W. Lake Ave.
Glenview, IL 60025
USA
Phone: 1-847-375-4715
Fax: 1-877-734-8758
International Fax: 1-732-460-7318
www.ampainsoc.org

The Arthritis Foundation
PO Box 7669
Atlanta, GA 30357
USA
Phone: 1-800-283-7800
www.arthritis.org

Bibliography

Chapter 1

American Geriatrics Society Panel on Chronic Pain in Older Persons. The management of chronic pain in older persons. *J Am Geriatr Soc* 1998; 46:635–651.

American Geriatrics Society Panel on Persistent Pain in Older Persons. The management of persistent pain in older persons. *J Am Geriatr Soc* 2002; 50:1–20.

Canadian Senate Standing Committee on Social Affairs, Science and Technology. *Quality End-of-Life Care: The Right of Every Canadian.* Available at: http://www.-parl.gc.ca/36/2/parlbus...m-e/upda-e/rep-e/repfinjun00.htm. Accessed July 16, 2001.

Charlton JE (Ed). *Core Curriculum for Professional Education in Pain*, 3rd ed. Seattle: IASP Press, 2005.

Cook A, Thomas M. Pain and the use of health services among the elderly. *J Aging Health* 1994; 6:155–174.

Ferrell BR, Novy D, Sullivan, MD, et al. Ethical dilemmas in pain management. *J Pain* 2001; 2:171–180.

Fisher R, Ross MR, MacLean MJ. *A Guide to End-of-Life Care for Seniors.* Ottawa: Health Canada, 2000.

Gibson SJ, Weiner DK (Eds). *Pain in Older Persons.* Seattle: IASP Press, 2005.

Millar WJ. Chronic pain. *Health Rep* 1996; 7:47–53.

Mobily PR, Herr KA, Clark MK, et al. An epidemiological analysis of pain in the elderly: the Iowa 65+ Rural Health Study. *J Aging Health* 1994; 62:139–154.

National Council on the Aging. *Facts about Older Americans and Pain.* Available at: http://ortho-mcneil.com/resources/misc/seniors_facts_bottom.htm. Accessed November 12, 2002.

Chapter 2

Caudill M, Schnable R, Zuttermeister P, et al. Decreased clinic use by chronic pain patients: response to behavioral medicine intervention. *Clin J Pain* 1991;7:305–310.

Hadjistavropoulos T, Craig KD (Eds). *Pain: Psychological Perspectives.* Mahwah, NJ: Lawrence Erlbaum Associates, 2004.

Hadjistavropoulos T, Herr K, Turk DC, et al. An interdisciplinary expert consensus statement on pain assessment in older persons. *Clin J Pain* 2007; 23:S1–S42.

Hale C, Hadjistavropoulos T. Emotional components of pain. *Pain Res Manage* 1997; 2:217–225.

Herr K. Pain assessment in the older adult with verbal communication skills. In: Weiner D, Gibson SG (Eds). *Pain in Older Persons.* Seattle: IASP Press, 2005, pp 111–133.

Kirschenbaum DS. Self-regulatory failure: a review with clinical implications. *Clin Psychol Rev* 1987; 7:77–104.

Lorig K, Fries JF. *The Arthritis Helpbook.* Cambridge, MA: Perseus, 2000.

Melzack R. The short-form McGill Pain Questionnaire. Pain 1987; 30:191–197.

Merskey H, Bogduk N. *Classification of Chronic Pain: Descriptions of Chronic Pain and Definitions of Pain Terms.* Seattle: IASP Press, 1994.

Turk DC, Gatchel RJ (Eds). *Psychological Approaches to Pain Management: A Practitioner's Handbook.* New York: Guilford Press, 2002.

Chapter 3

Beck AT, Rush AJ, Shaw BF, et al. *Cognitive Therapy for Depression.* New York: Guilford Press, 1979.

Benson H. *The Relaxation Response.* New York: Morrow, 1976.

Bortz WM II. Disuse and aging. *JAMA* 1982; 248:1203–1208.

Burns D. *The Feeling Good Handbook.* New York: Plume, 1999.

Ellis A. *Rational Emotive Behavior Therapy: It Works for Me—It Can Work for You.* Amherst, NY: Prometheus, 2004.

National Institutes of Health Technology Assessment Panel. Integration of behavioral and relaxation approaches into the treatment of chronic pain and insomnia. *JAMA* 1996; 276:313–318.

Turk DC, Winter F. *The Pain Survival Guide: How to Reclaim Your Life.* Washington, DC: APA, 2004.

Chapter 4

Beck AT, Rush AJ, Shaw BF, et al. *Cognitive Therapy for Depression.* New York: Guilford Press, 1979.

Burns D. *The Feeling Good Handbook.* New York: Plume, 1999.

Corey D. Pain: *Learning to Live Without It.* Toronto: Macmillan, 1993, pp 130–134.

Cousins N. *Anatomy of An Illness.* New York: Norton, 1979.

Engel J. *The Complete Canadian Health Guide.* Toronto: Key Porter, 2005, pp 401–405.

Lewinsohn PM, Munoz R, Youngren, MA, et al. *Control Your Depression.* New York: Fireside, 1992.

Lorig K, Fries, JF. *The Arthritis Helpbook,* 5th ed. Cambridge, MA: Perseus, 2000.

Waters SJ, Woodward JT, Keefe FJ. Cognitive-behavioral therapy for pain in older adults. In: Weiner D, Gibson SG (Eds). *Pain in Older Persons.* Seattle: IASP Press, 2005, pp 239–261.

Chapter 5

Hall M, Havens B. Social isolation and social loneliness. In: *Writings in Gerontology: Mental Health and Aging.* Ottawa: National Advisory Council on Aging, 2002, pp 33–42.

Jacobs JM, Hammerman-Rozenberg R, Cohen A, et al. Chronic back pain among the elderly: prevalence, associations and predictors. *Spine* 2006; 31:E203–E207.

Lauder W, Mummery K, Jones M, et al. A comparison of health behaviours in lonely and non-lonely populations. *Psychol Health Med* 2006; 11:233–245.

Schultz NR, Moore D. Loneliness: Correlates, attributions and coping among older adults. *Pers Soc Psychol Bull* 1984; 10:67–77.

Waltz M, Kriegel W, van't Pad Bosch, P. The social environment and health in rheumatoid arthritis: marital quality predicts individual variability in pain severity. *Arthritis Care Res* 1998; 11:356–374.

Chapter 6

American Geriatrics Society. Exercise prescription for older adults with osteoarthritis pain: consensus practice recommendations. *J Am Geriatr Soc* 2001; 49:808–823.

Binkley JM, Stratford PW, Lott SA, et al. The Lower Extremity Functional Scale (LEFS): scale development, measurement properties, and clinical application. *Phys Ther* 1999; 79:371–383.

Borg G. Perceived exertion as indicator of somatic stress. *Scand J Rehabil Med* 1970; 2:92–98.

Corey D. Pain: *Learning to Live Without It.* Toronto: Macmillan, 1993.

Cotman CW, Engesser-Cesar C. Exercise enhances and protects brain function. *Exerc Sport Sci* Rev 2002; 30:75–79.

Heart and Stroke Foundation Canada. *Fitness on the Run.* Ottawa: Heart Smart Fitness Program, Heart and Stroke Foundation, 2000.

Hurley O. *Safe Therapeutic Exercise for the Frail Elderly: An Introduction* (2nd ed). Albany, NY: Center for the Study of Aging, 1996.

President's Proposed Drug Relief Plan Must Include Relief from America's Worst Ailment: Physical Inactivity. Available at: http://www.ncpad.org. Accessed June 20, 2007.

Rikli R, Jones J. *Senior Fitness Test Manual.* Human Kinetics, 2001.

Shephard RJ. *Aging, Physical Activity and Health.* Windsor: Human Kinetics, 1997.

Chapter 7

Alexander NB, Koester DJ, Grunawalt JA. Chair design affects how older adults rise from a chair. *J Am Geriatr Soc* 1996; 44: 356–362.

Arthritis Society. The Arthritis *Society Pages Tips for Living Well and Exercising Regularly.* Available at: http://www.arthritis.ca/tips%20for%20living/default.asp?s=1. Accessed June 20, 2007.

Brach JS, VanSwearingen JM. Physical impairment and disability: relationship to performance of activities of daily living in community-dwelling older men. *Phys Ther* 2002; 82:752–761.

Buszewicz M, Rait G, Griffen M, et al. Self management of arthritis in primary care: randomized controlled trial. *BMJ* 2006; 333:879.

Helewa A, Walker JM. *Physical Therapy in Arthritis.* Oxford: W.B. Saunders, 1996.

Mann WC, Hurren D, Tomita M. Assistive devices used by home-based elderly persons with arthritis. *Am J Occup Ther* 1995; 49:810–820.

Pitt-Nairn EJ, Relf PE, McDaniel AR. Analysis of factors which can affect the preferences of older individuals for hand pruners. *Phys Occup Ther Geriatr* 1992; 10:77–90.

Pinto MR, De Medici S, Alotnicki A, et al. Reduced visual acuity in elderly people: the role of ergonomics and gerontechnology. *Age Ageing* 1997; 26:339–344.

Puniello MS, McGibbon C, Krebs DE. Lifting strategy and stability in strength-impaired elders. *Spine* 2001; 26:731–737.

Schultz-Larsen K, Aylund K. Tiredness in daily activities: A subjective measure for the identification of frailty among non-disabled community-living older adults. *Arch Gerontol Geriatr* 2007; 44:83–93.

Chapter 8

Ancoli-Israel S, Poceta JS, Stepnowsky C, et al. Identification and treatment of sleep problems in the elderly. *Sleep Med Rev* 1997; 1:3–17.

Bales C, Ritchie C. *Handbook of Clinical Nutrition and Aging.* Totowa, NJ: Humana Press, 2004.

Dietary Guidelines Advisory Committee. *Dietary Guidelines for Americans,* 6th ed. Washington, DC: U.S. Government Printing Office, 2005.

Division of Aging and Seniors. *Nutrition and Healthy Aging.* Available at: http://www.phac-aspc.gc.ca/seniors-aines/pubs/workshop_healthyaging/nutrition/nutrition1_e.htm. Accessed March 8, 2007.

Foley D, Ancoli-Israel S, Britz P, et al. Sleep disturbances and chronic disease in older adults: results of the 2003 National Sleep Foundation Sleep in America Study. *J Psychosom Res* 2004; 56:497–502.

Health Canada. *Eating Well with Canada's Food Guide.* Ottawa: Minister of Public Works and Government Services Canada, 2007.

Hoffman S. Sleep in the older adult: implications for nurses. *Geriatr Nurs* 2003; 24:210–216.

Lacks P. *Behavioral Treatment for Persistent Insomnia.* New York: Elsevier, 1987.

Larson Duyff R. *Complete Food and Nutrition Guide,* 2nd ed. Hoboken, NJ: American Dietetic Association, 2002.

Niedert K, Dorner B. *Nutrition Care of the Older Adult: A Handbook for Registered Dietitians Working Throughout the Continuum of Care,* 2nd ed. Chicago: American Dietetic Association, 2005.

Public Health Agency of Canada. What are sleeping pills and tranquillizers? Available at: http://www.phac-aspc.gc.ca/seniors-aines/pubs/sleeping_tranq/seniors_sleep/seniors_sleeping_1e.htm. Accessed February 4, 2007.

Chapter 9

Caring Connections. How to talk to your doctor about pain. Available at: http://www.caringinfo.org/i4a/pages/index.cfm?pageid=3478. Accessed January 12, 2007.

Galloway J. How we tell our doctor about pain. *N Y State Med* 1991; 91:399–400.

Goldman B. Chronic pain patients must cope with chronic lack of physician understanding. *CMAJ* 1991; 144:1493–1497.

Manitoba Health and Manitoba Seniors Secretariat. Questions to ask your doctor and pharmacist. Available at: http://www.gov.mb.ca/shas/pdf/questions_05.pdf . Accessed January 12, 2007.

Stewart M, Roter D. *Communicating with Medical Patients.* Newbury Park, CA: Sage Publications, 1989.

Chapter 10

National Council on the Aging. *The Pain & Older Americans Survey.* Conducted by Louis Harris & Associates, 1997.

National Academy on an Aging Society. *Challenges for the 21st Century: Chronic and Disabling Conditions,* No. 3. Washington, DC: National Academy on an Aging Society, 2000.

Heffernan JJ. Low back. In: Noble J, Greene II HL, Modest GA et al. (Eds). *Textbook of Primary Care Medicine* (2nd ed). St. Louis: Mosby, 1996, pp 1026–1040.

Lorig K, Fries JF. *The Arthritis Helpbook,* 5th ed. Cambridge, MA: Perseus, 2000.

Merskey H, Bogduk N. *Classification of Chronic Pain: Descriptions of Chronic Pain Syndromes and Definitions of Pain Terms,* 2nd ed. Seattle: IASP Press, 1994.

Millar WJ. Chronic pain. *Health Rep* 1996; 7:47–53.

Resnick N, Dosa D. Geriatric medicine. In Kasper DL (Ed), *Harrison's Principles of Internal Medicine,* 16th ed. New York: McGraw-Hill, 2005.

Stein WM. Cancer pain in the elderly. In Ferrell BR, Ferrell BA (Eds). *Pain in the Elderly.* Seattle: IASP Press, 1996, pp 69–80.

Thomas J, von Gunten C. Clinical management of dyspnea. *Lancet Oncol* 2002; 3:223–228.

Vestergaard K, Andersen G, Jensen TS. Central post-stroke pain. In Crombie IK, Croft PR, Linton SJ et al. (Eds). *Epidemiology of Pain.* Seattle: IASP Press, 1999, pp 155–158.

Webster L, Webster R. Predicting aberrant behaviors in opioid-treated patients: preliminary validation of the opioid risk tool. *Pain Med* 2005; 6:432–442.

Chapter 11

American Psychiatric Association. Practice guideline for the treatment of patients with Alzheimer's disease and other dementias of late life. Available at: http://www.psych.org/psych_pract/treatg/quick_ref_guide/AlzheimersQRG_04-15-05.pdf. Accessed March 26, 2007.

Cohen CA, Colantonio A, Vernich L. Positive aspects of caregiving: rounding out the caregiver experience. *Int J Geriatr Psychiatry* 2002; 17:184–188.

Corey D. Pain: *Learning to Live Without It*. Toronto: Macmillan, 1993.

Feldt KS. The checklist of nonverbal pain indicators. *Pain Manag Nurs* 2000; 1:13–21.

Fuchs-Lacelle S, Hadjistavropoulos T. Development and preliminary validation of the Pain Assessment Checklist for Seniors with Limited Ability to Communicate (PACSLAC). *Pain Manag Nurs* 2004; 5:37–49.

Shephard RJ. *Aging, Physical Activity and Health*. Champaign, IL: Human Kinetics, 1997.

Zwakhalen SM, Hamers JP, Berger MP. The psychometric quality and clinical usefulness of three pain assessment tools for elderly people with dementia. *Pain* 2006; 126:210–220.

Index

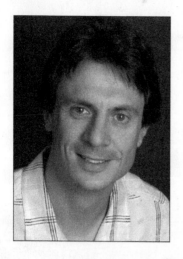

Thomas Hadjistavropoulos, PhD, RD Psych, is Professor of Clinical Psychology and Director of the Centre on Aging and Health, University of Regina, Canada. Together with his graduate students and collaborators, he has dedicated the last 16 years to investigating better ways of assessing and managing pain among older persons. He has received the Canadian Institutes of Health Research Career Investigator Award, a Saskatchewan Health Research Foundation Achievement Award, a Canadian Pain Society Early Career Award, a Saskatchewan Health Care Excellence Award for Innovation, a Saskatchewan Centennial Medal, a University of Regina Research Excellence Award, and other distinctions. He has also been elected fellow of the Canadian Psychological Association in recognition of distinguished contributions to the science and profession of psychology.

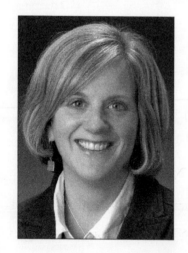

Heather D. Hadjistavropoulos, PhD, RD Psych, is Professor of Psychology and Director of Clinical Psychology Training at the University of Regina. She founded the Psychology Training Clinic at the university and developed a state-of-the-art Clinical Health Psychology Area for research, teaching, and practice. Her research is of direct relevance to older persons and focuses on understanding and improving the quality of health care in an attempt to reduce the burden of illness, as well as on assessing and treating psychological problems that have an impact on health. She has published and presented her research widely and has received funding through the Canadian Health Services Research Foundation and Canadian Institute of Health Research. She has been awarded the Canadian Psychological Association's President's New Researcher Award, the Canadian Pain Society's Early Career Award, the YWCA Woman of Distinction (Health and Wellness), the University of Regina's Research Excellence Award, and the University of Regina's President's Scholar Award.